MASTERING REFLEXOLOGY

Relieve Stress, Boost Wellness, and Master the Technique

Dr. Trent EM

Copyright Page© Dr. Trent EM 2024

Table of Contents

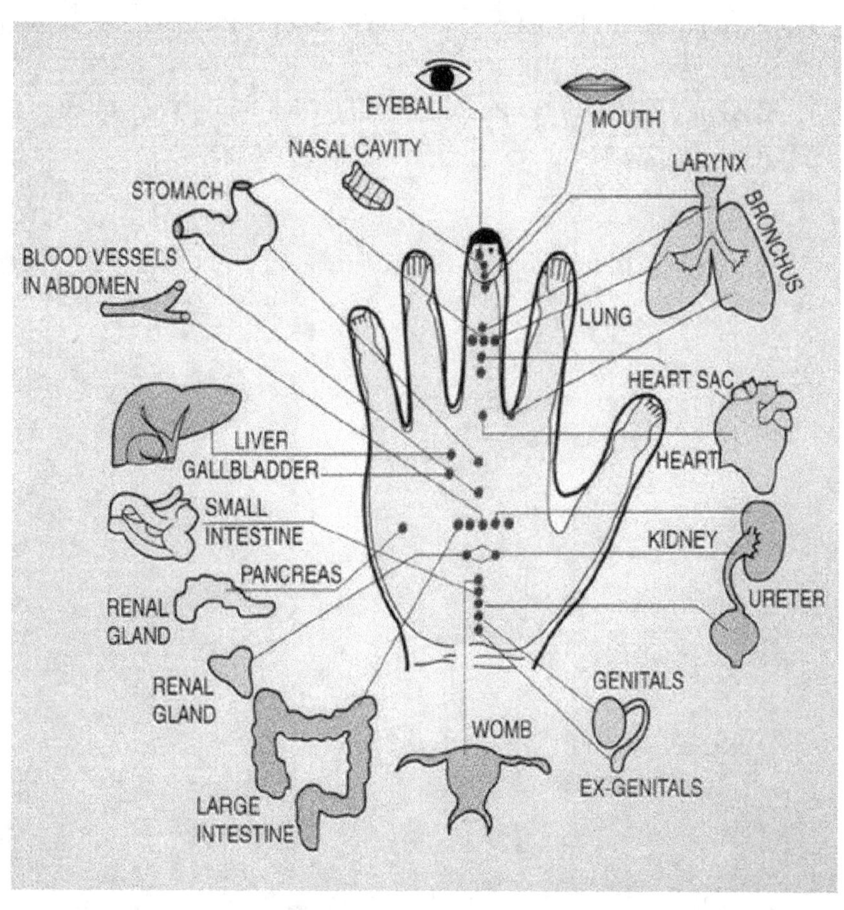
EYEBALL
MOUTH
NASAL CAVITY
LARYNX
STOMACH
BRONCHUS
BLOOD VESSELS
IN ABDOMEN
LUNG
HEART SAC
LIVER
GALLBLADDER
HEART
SMALL
INTESTINE
KIDNEY
PANCREAS
RENAL
GLAND
URETER
RENAL
GLAND
GENITALS
WOMB
EX-GENITALS
LARGE
INTESTINE

Introduction

A Walk in the Park... on Your Feet!

Have you ever stopped to truly appreciate your feet? They carry you through life, silently enduring countless miles. Yet, when was the last time you treated them (and yourself) to a truly rejuvenating experience? Reflexology offers a unique path to well-being, one that starts with a simple step – literally.

This book isn't just about pampering your feet (although that's certainly a welcome perk!). It's about unlocking an ancient practice with the power to reduce stress, improve your mood, and enhance your overall health.

Think of this book as your personal guide to the fascinating world of reflexology. Within these pages, you'll discover:

- The history and science behind reflexology – how this ancient practice has stood the test of time.

- A detailed map of your body, revealed through your feet, hands, and even ears!

- Easy-to-follow techniques you can use to give yourself or a loved one a relaxing and therapeutic reflexology session.

- The incredible benefits of reflexology, from stress reduction and improved sleep to pain management and a stronger immune system.

- Whether reflexology is right for you, and how to find a qualified practitioner if you'd prefer someone else to do the walking (on your reflexology map, that is!).

By the end of this journey, you'll be equipped with the knowledge and tools to take control of your well-being, one step at a time. So, put on your comfiest socks, grab a cup of tea, and get ready to explore the incredible world of reflexology. You might be surprised at what your feet have to tell you!

What is Reflexology and How Does it Work? (Unveiling the Ancient Secret)

Reflexology, a practice with roots stretching back thousands of years, offers a unique approach to promoting relaxation and potentially improving overall health. But what exactly is it, and how does it work? Let's delve into the fascinating world of reflexology and unveil the ancient secret behind this touch therapy.

The Theory Behind the Touch

Reflexology is based on the principle that specific reflex points on the feet, hands, ears, and even face correspond to various organs and systems within the body. By applying gentle pressure or massage techniques to these reflex points, practitioners aim to stimulate a healing response in the corresponding areas.

There are two main schools of thought on how reflexology might work:

- **The Nervous System Connection:** One theory suggests that applying pressure to reflex points sends signals through the nervous system, potentially promoting relaxation, improving circulation, and influencing the body's natural healing mechanisms.

- **The Energy Pathway Theory:** Another theory, rooted in traditional Chinese medicine, proposes that reflexology works by stimulating the flow of vital energy (qi) throughout the body. By balancing this energy flow, reflexology may help restore harmony and promote well-being.

The Historical Roots

The exact origins of reflexology remain shrouded in some mystery. Evidence suggests practices similar to reflexology existed in ancient Egypt, China, and other civilizations. However, the term "reflexology" itself emerged in the early 20th century, pioneered by Eunice Ingham in the United States and Doreen Bailey in the United Kingdom.

Modern Applications

While scientific studies on the effectiveness of reflexology are ongoing, many people swear by its benefits. It's often used as a complementary therapy alongside conventional medicine to help manage:

- Stress and anxiety

- Pain, including headaches and migraines

- Digestive issues

- Sleep problems

- And more

It's important to remember that reflexology is not a substitute for medical care. However, it can be a valuable tool for relaxation and potentially enhancing overall well-being when used in conjunction with traditional treatments.

Your First Steps into Reflexology

The beauty of reflexology lies in its simplicity and accessibility. Unlike some massage therapies, it doesn't require elaborate equipment or expensive oils. With a basic understanding of the reflex points and a gentle touch, you can begin exploring the potential benefits of reflexology for yourself.

This book will be your guide as you unveil the secrets of reflexology. We'll explore detailed reflexology maps, teach you effective techniques, and delve deeper into the potential benefits this ancient practice offers. So, get ready to embark on a journey of discovery – a journey that starts with a touch and leads to a path of relaxation and potential wellness.

Stepping onto the Path of Reflexology: What to Expect and How to Get Started

Curious about exploring reflexology but unsure where to begin? Don't worry, here you will be equiped with the knowledge you need to take your first steps on this path to potential relaxation and wellness.

What to Expect During a Reflexology Session

Your first reflexology session will likely involve a conversation with the practitioner. They'll ask about your overall health, any specific concerns you might have, and any medications you're taking. This helps them tailor the session to your individual needs.

Setting the Stage for Relaxation

The environment typically promotes relaxation. Many practitioners use calming music, soft lighting, and comfortable seating or tables. You'll likely be asked to remove your shoes and socks, and some practitioners might use lotion or oil to facilitate smoother hand and foot movements.

The Art of Touch

The reflexology practitioner will then gently apply pressure to specific reflex points on your feet, hands, ears, or face, depending on the chosen approach. The pressure should be firm but comfortable, never painful.

Some people experience a tingling sensation or even mild discomfort in certain areas, but this typically subsides quickly.

The Power of Relaxation

Many people find reflexology sessions deeply relaxing. It's common to feel a sense of calm wash over you, and some people even drift off to sleep during the session.

What to Expect After Your Session

After your reflexology session, you might feel energized or more relaxed. Some people experience temporary detoxification symptoms like increased urination or thirst. These are generally mild and pass quickly. Drinking plenty of water throughout the day can help your body flush out any toxins released during the session.

Getting Started with Reflexology

Here are some tips to help you get started with reflexology:

- **Find a qualified practitioner:** Look for reflexologists certified by a reputable organization. Ask for recommendations from friends, family, or your doctor.

- **Communicate openly:** Discuss your health history and any concerns you have with the practitioner before your session. Let them know if you experience any discomfort during the session.

- **Be patient and consistent:** Like any therapy, reflexology works best with regular sessions. While some people experience immediate benefits, others may need a few sessions to feel the full effect.

- **Listen to your body:** Pay attention to how you feel after a session. If you experience any concerning side effects, reach out to your healthcare provider.

Reflexology at Home

While a professional reflexology session offers a tailored approach, you can also explore self-reflexology at home. This book will provide detailed reflexology charts and instructions on basic techniques you can practice on yourself or loved ones.

Remember, reflexology is a journey of self-discovery and potential well-being. By taking the first step and exploring this ancient practice, you're opening yourself to a world of relaxation and a renewed sense of balance.

Part 1:
The Reflexology Map - Charting Your Course to Wellness

13

Chapter 1:

Understanding the Reflexology Zones

Demystifying the Foot Map (illustrated with a detailed reflexology foot chart)

The human foot, often relegated to simply supporting our weight, holds a hidden map – a map to our entire well-being according to the principles of reflexology. By understanding and applying pressure to specific reflex points on the feet, we can potentially influence the corresponding organs and systems within the body.

This section will be your guide to deciphering this fascinating foot map, equipping you with the knowledge to unlock the potential of reflexology.

Decoding the Map: A Zone-by-Zone Breakdown

As you look at the reflexology foot chart, you'll notice various zones corresponding to different parts of the body. Let's delve into some key areas:

- **The Toes:** The big toe reflexology zone is believed to correspond to the head and brain. The other toes represent various facial features and sinuses.

- **The Ball of the Foot:** This area generally maps to the upper body organs, including the lungs, heart, and stomach.

- **The Arch:** The arch of the foot is often associated with the digestive system, including the liver, intestines, and colon.

- **The Heel:** The heel reflexology zone typically reflects the lower body, including the bladder, kidneys, and reproductive organs.

A Detailed Look at the Reflexology Foot Chart

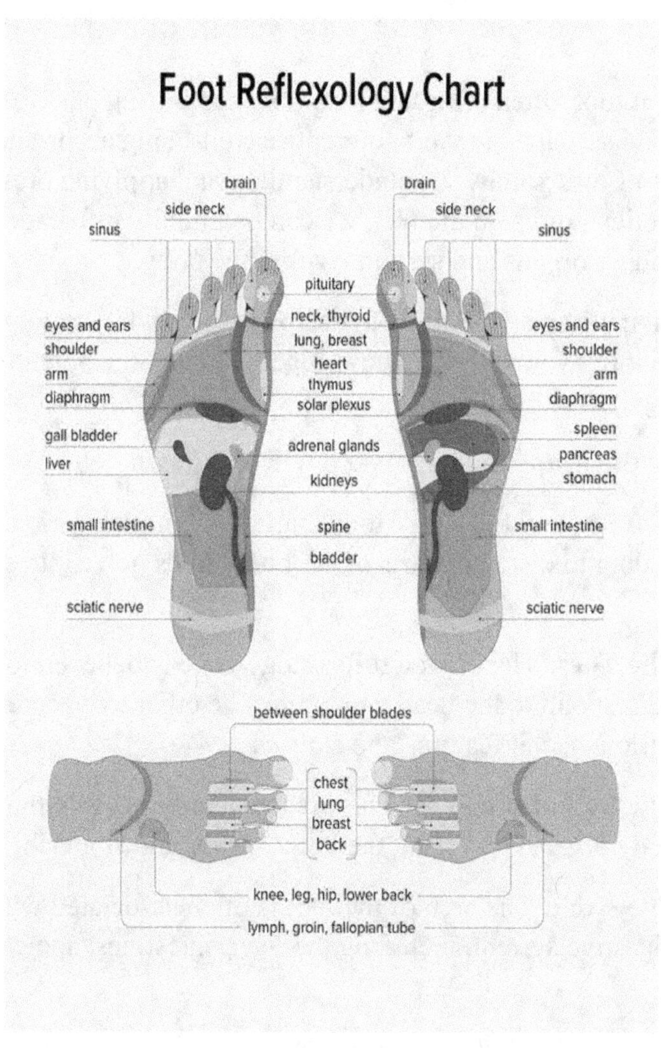

Understanding the Pressure Points

Each zone on the foot chart is further divided into smaller reflex points, each believed to correspond to a specific organ or system. These reflex points may feel slightly tender or bumpy when pressed.

Here are some general guidelines for applying pressure to these points:

- **Use your thumb or index finger:** These fingers offer the most control and pressure variation.

- **Apply gentle but firm pressure:** Aim for a comfortable intensity that allows you to feel a slight indentation but doesn't cause pain.

- **Hold for a few seconds:** Maintain pressure for 3-5 seconds before releasing.

- **Repeat on both feet:** Reflexology is typically practiced on both feet, as each foot is believed to mirror the entire body.

Remember: This is just a general overview. The specific location and pressure used for each reflex point may vary slightly depending on the reflexology chart you're referencing.

Beyond the Basics:

The reflexology foot chart serves as a valuable starting point. However, as you gain experience, you can explore more nuanced techniques. For instance, some practitioners use specific stroking or walking motions on the foot to stimulate reflex points.

Unlocking the Power of the Foot Map

By understanding the reflexology zones and applying gentle pressure to specific points, you can potentially:

- **Promote relaxation and reduce stress:** Focusing on the feet and applying pressure can trigger the body's relaxation response.

- **Improve circulation:** Reflexology may help stimulate blood flow throughout the body, potentially aiding in the delivery of oxygen and nutrients.

- **Support overall well-being:** By addressing specific reflex points, you might target areas of concern and promote a sense of balance and well-being.

Remember: Reflexology is a complementary therapy, not a replacement for medical care. Always consult your doctor before starting any new therapy, especially if you have any underlying health conditions.

This detailed exploration of the reflexology foot chart equips you with the foundational knowledge to begin your reflexology journey. As you delve deeper into this practice, you'll discover the power held within the often-overlooked map etched on your feet.

A Handy Guide to Hand Reflexology (including a clear hand reflexology chart)

While the feet are often the primary focus in reflexology, the hands also hold a wealth of potential for promoting relaxation and well-being. This section will equip you with the knowledge to explore the fascinating map of reflexology on your hands, providing a convenient and accessible way to experience the benefits of this practice.

The Hand Reflexology Map: A Universe at Your Fingertips

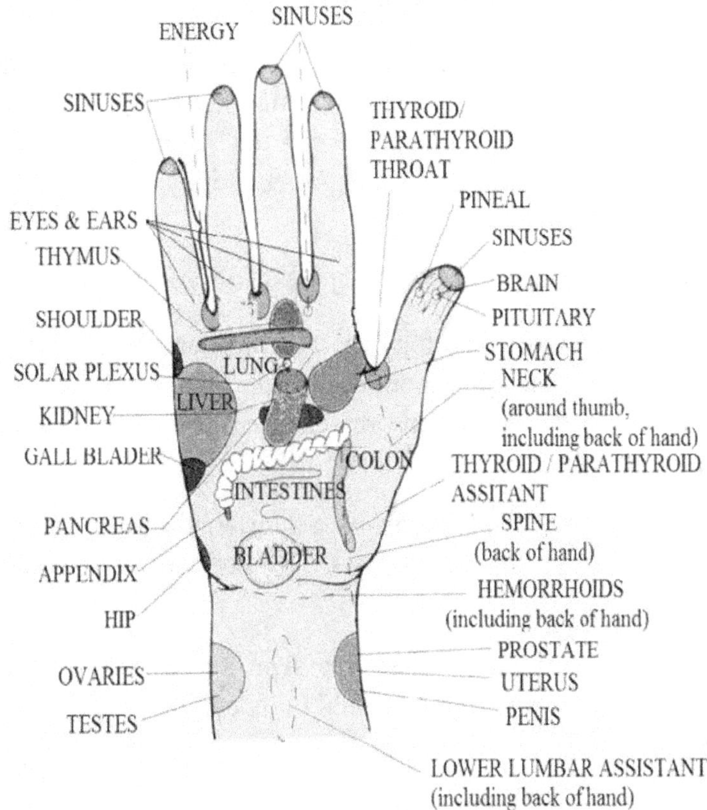

Decoding the Hand Map: A Zone-by-Zone Exploration

Just like the feet, our hands offer a microcosm of the entire body through reflexology. Here's a breakdown of some key areas:

- **The Thumb:** The thumb reflexology zone is believed to correspond to the head and brain.

- **The Fingers:** Each finger is associated with different organs. The index finger often reflects the spine, the middle finger the digestive system, the ring finger the urinary system, and the pinky finger the heart and lungs.

- **The Palm:** The palm generally maps to the lower body and torso. The fleshy area at the base of the thumb can represent the chest and lungs, while the center of the palm reflects the digestive system. The wrist area often corresponds to the reproductive organs.

Exploring the Reflex Points

Similar to the foot, the hand reflexology chart showcases specific reflex points believed to influence corresponding organs. These points may feel slightly tender or textured when pressed. Here are some general guidelines for applying pressure:

- **Use your thumb, index finger, or a gentle rubbing motion:** The smaller size of the hand allows for more delicate pressure application.

- **Apply gentle but firm pressure:** Aim for a comfortable intensity that allows you to feel a slight indentation but doesn't cause pain.

- **Hold for a few seconds:** Maintain pressure for 3-5 seconds before releasing.

- **Work both hands:** Reflexology is typically practiced on both hands, mirroring the effect on the whole body.

The Benefits of Hand Reflexology

Hand reflexology offers several advantages:

- **Convenience:** Your hands are readily available, making it easy to incorporate reflexology into your daily routine.

- **Portability:** You can practice hand reflexology on yourself or even offer a brief session to a friend or family member while traveling or waiting in line.

- **Focus on Specific Areas:** Since the hand map is more compact, you can easily target a specific area of concern, such as the head or digestive system, by focusing on the corresponding reflex points.

Considerations for Hand Reflexology

While generally safe, there are a few things to keep in mind:

- **Avoid applying pressure to swollen, injured, or inflamed areas of the hand.**

- **If you have any underlying health conditions, consult your doctor before starting hand reflexology.**

Unlocking the Potential of Your Hands

By understanding the reflexology zones on your hands and applying gentle pressure to specific points, you can potentially:

- **Reduce stress and anxiety:** Focusing on the hands and applying pressure can promote relaxation and a sense of calm.

- **Improve sleep quality:** Stimulating certain reflex points on the hands may promote better sleep patterns.

- **Alleviate headaches:** Applying pressure to specific reflex points on the hand may help ease tension headaches.

A Handy Companion on Your Reflexology Journey

The hand reflexology chart acts as your guide to exploring the world of reflexology within your own hands. This convenient and accessible approach allows you to experience the potential benefits of reflexology anytime, anywhere. As you delve deeper into this practice, you'll discover the power held within your fingertips, waiting to be unlocked through the gentle touch of reflexology.

Exploring Additional Reflexology Zones: Ear, Face, and Beyond (with illustrative diagrams)

The world of reflexology extends beyond the well-known maps of the feet and hands. While these zones offer a powerful gateway to well-being, venturing into other reflexology areas can provide even more options for promoting relaxation and potentially addressing specific concerns.

The Microuniverse of the Ear: Auricular Reflexology

The ear, often seen as simply the organ of hearing, holds a surprisingly detailed reflexology map according to some practitioners. This map, known as auricular reflexology, proposes that specific points on the outer ear correspond to various organs and systems within the body.

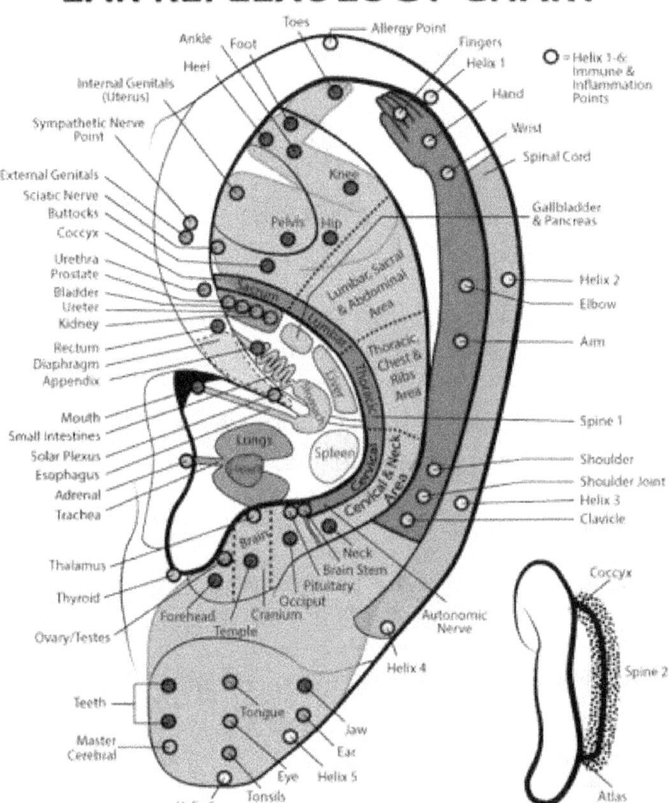

Exploring the Ear Map:

While the specific location of reflex points may vary slightly depending on the chart, some general zones include:

- **The Earlobe:** This area often reflects the head and brain.

- **The Upper Cartilage:** Points along the upper ridge of the ear may correspond to the lungs and digestive system.

- **The Central Cartilage:** This area might hold reflex points for the heart, spine, and reproductive organs.

Applying Pressure on the Ear:

When working with the ear, it's crucial to use a gentle touch due to its delicate nature. Here are some guidelines:

- **Use your thumb and index finger:** gently pinch or hold specific reflex points.

- **Apply very light pressure:** Aim for a barely-there pressure that doesn't cause any discomfort.

- **Hold for a few seconds:** Similar to other reflexology techniques, maintain pressure for 3-5 seconds before releasing.

- **Work both ears:** Reflexology is typically practiced on both ears, as each is believed to mirror the entire body.

Important Considerations:

- Auricular reflexology is not recommended for people with ear infections, open wounds, or implanted devices in the ear.

- As with other reflexology practices, consult your doctor before starting auricular reflexology, especially if you have any underlying health conditions.

The Face: A Map of Expression and Well-being

Facial reflexology delves into the connection between pressure points on the face and their potential influence on internal organs and emotions. By applying gentle pressure to specific areas of the face, practitioners aim to promote relaxation, address specific concerns, and even enhance emotional well-being.

[Insert an illustration of a detailed facial reflexology chart here. The chart should clearly label the reflex points for major organs and body systems on the face.]

Exploring the Facial Map:

The facial reflexology map can be quite intricate, but here are some key areas:

- **The Eyebrows:** These areas might correspond to the head, sinuses, and digestive system.

- **The Bridge of the Nose:** This point is often associated with the lungs and heart.

- **The Cheeks:** Reflex points on the cheeks may connect to the stomach, intestines, and immune system.

Applying Pressure on the Face:

Similar to the ear, a gentle touch is crucial when working with the face. Here's what to keep in mind:

- **Use your fingertips:** Lightly press or tap on specific reflex points.

- **Apply very light pressure:** Maintain a pressure that feels comfortable and doesn't cause any irritation.

- **Hold for a few seconds:** Similar to other reflexology techniques, hold pressure for 3-5 seconds before releasing.

- **Focus on areas of concern:** You can target specific facial areas based on your needs, such as the temples for headaches or the brow line for sinus congestion.

Important Considerations:

- Avoid applying pressure to the eyes or any areas with open wounds or blemishes.

- As always, consult your doctor before starting facial reflexology, especially if you have any underlying skin conditions.

Beyond the Feet, Hands, Ears, and Face

The world of reflexology extends even further. Some practitioners explore reflexology zones on the head, neck, and even the torso. While these areas may be less commonly used, they offer additional options for a truly holistic approach.

A World of Possibilities

By venturing beyond the well-known reflexology maps, you unlock a wider range of possibilities for promoting relaxation, potentially addressing specific concerns, and enhancing overall well-being. Remember, the key is to start slowly, experiment with different zones, and always prioritize comfort and safety.

This exploration of additional reflexology zones equips you with the knowledge to expand your practice and potentially unlock a deeper level of well-being. As you delve into these fascinating microcosms within your body, you'll discover the vast potential that reflexology holds.

Chapter 2:

Reading the Body's Story Through Your Feet

Foot Assessment: What Your Feet Can Tell You About Your Health

The human foot, often relegated to supporting our weight and navigating the world, holds a hidden language. According to the principles of reflexology, the condition of your feet can offer valuable clues about your overall health and well-being. By learning to "read" your feet, you can gain valuable insights and potentially identify areas that might benefit from reflexology or other complementary therapies.

Foot Assessment: A Window into Your Health

Here's how to conduct a simple foot assessment at home:

- **Gather Your Supplies:** All you need is a well-lit space and a mirror for a good look at the soles of your feet.

- **Observe the Overall Appearance:** Start by looking at the general condition of your feet. Are there any cracks, calluses, or discoloration? These can sometimes indicate areas of dryness, pressure overload, or potential imbalances.

- **Feel the Temperature:** Are your feet generally warm or cold? Cold feet could be a sign of poor circulation, while excessively hot feet might suggest inflammation.

- **Assess Flexibility:** Try gently bending and flexing your toes. Are there any limitations in movement or areas that feel stiff? Reduced flexibility might indicate tension or potential joint issues.

- **Check for Tenderness:** Gently press on different areas of your foot. Are there any specific points that feel particularly tender or painful? These areas might correspond to reflex points associated with organs or systems that could benefit from attention.

Foot Characteristics and Potential Meanings

While it's important to remember that foot assessment is not a definitive diagnosis, here are some general associations to consider:

- **Dry, Cracked Heels:** This could indicate dehydration or a vitamin deficiency.

- **Calluses:** These often form in areas of repetitive pressure and friction. They might point to improper footwear or gait issues.

- **Bunions and Hammertoes:** These bony deformities can be caused by tight-fitting shoes or underlying conditions.

- **Swollen Ankles:** This could be a sign of fluid retention, poor circulation, or even an allergic reaction.

- **Cold Feet:** This might indicate poor circulation or a sluggish metabolism.

- **Hot Feet:** This could suggest inflammation, hormonal changes, or even nerve damage.

Important Considerations:

- **Don't Self-Diagnose:** If you notice any concerning signs or symptoms during your foot assessment, consult your doctor for a proper diagnosis and treatment plan.

- **Listen to Your Body:** Pain or discomfort in your feet is a signal to pay attention. Consider modifying your footwear, addressing any underlying health issues, or seeking professional help.

- **Reflexology is a Complementary Therapy:** Foot assessment can be a valuable tool, but it should not replace medical advice or treatment.

Using Foot Assessment to Enhance Your Reflexology Practice

By understanding what your feet are telling you, you can tailor your reflexology sessions for optimal benefit:

- **Target Specific Areas:** If your foot assessment reveals tenderness in a specific reflex zone, you can focus on applying pressure to that area during your reflexology session.

- **Monitor Progress:** Regular foot assessment can help you track the impact of your reflexology practice. Over time, you might notice improvements in flexibility, reduced tenderness, or even a change in overall foot temperature.

- **Identify Underlying Issues:** Foot assessment can sometimes reveal signs that warrant discussing with your doctor. Early detection of potential problems can lead to timely intervention and better health outcomes.

Common Foot Reflexology Signs and Their Meanings

As you embark on your reflexology journey, your feet will become more than just tools for getting around. They'll transform into a map, potentially revealing clues about your overall well-being through various signs. Here's a guide to some common foot reflexology signs and their possible meanings:

Tenderness:

- **Location:** Tenderness in a specific reflex point on your foot might indicate an imbalance or potential sluggishness in the corresponding organ or system.

- **Meaning:** For example, tenderness in the ball of the foot, where the lung reflex zone is located, could suggest a predisposition to respiratory issues or simply indicate that you might benefit from deeper breaths throughout the day.

- **Action:** Focus on applying gentle pressure to the tender area during your reflexology session. You can also explore complementary practices like breathing exercises or consider consulting your doctor if the tenderness persists.

Calluses:

- **Location:** Calluses typically form on areas of your feet that experience repeated pressure and friction.

- **Meaning:** Their presence might suggest improper footwear or gait issues that could be contributing to the discomfort.

- **Action:** Evaluate your footwear and ensure it provides proper support and cushioning. Consider consulting a podiatrist or physical therapist for guidance on correcting any gait imbalances.

Dryness and Cracked Heels:

- **Location:** Dry, cracked heels are a common sign of dehydration or potential vitamin deficiencies.

- **Meaning:** This dryness can indicate a lack of essential moisture in your body, potentially impacting the health of your skin.

- **Action:** Increase your water intake and consider using a nourishing foot cream to address the dryness. A balanced diet rich in vitamins and minerals can also be beneficial.

Cold Feet:

- **Location:** Consistently cold feet can be a sign of poor circulation or a sluggish metabolism.

- **Meaning:** Cold feet might indicate that your body is struggling to efficiently deliver warm blood throughout your extremities.

- **Action:** Regular exercise can help improve circulation. Warming socks or a footbath can provide temporary relief. Consult your doctor if chronic cold feet persist, as they could indicate an underlying condition.

Sweaty Feet:

- **Location:** Excessive sweating in your feet can be caused by various factors, including stress, hormonal changes, or even certain medications.

- **Meaning:** Sweaty feet can create an environment conducive to fungal infections.

- **Action:** Wear breathable shoes and socks made from natural fibers like cotton or wool. Maintaining good foot hygiene and regularly changing your socks can help manage moisture levels. Consult your doctor if excessive sweating persists or is accompanied by other concerning symptoms.

Swollen Ankles:

- **Location:** Swollen ankles can be caused by fluid retention, poor circulation, or even an allergic reaction.

- **Meaning:** Swelling can indicate that excess fluid is accumulating in your tissues.

- **Action:** Reduce your sodium intake and elevate your feet when resting. If the swelling is sudden, severe, or accompanied by other symptoms like redness or pain, consult your doctor immediately.

Remember:

- These are general interpretations, and the meaning of a specific foot reflexology sign can vary depending on individual circumstances.

- It's important to consult your doctor if you experience any persistent or concerning signs in your feet.

- Reflexology should be a complementary therapy, not a substitute for medical care.

Paying attention to these common foot reflexology signs, you can gain valuable insights into your overall health. Remember, your feet are a vital part of your body, constantly communicating with you. Understanding their language, you can use reflexology and other self-care practices to address potential imbalances and promote well-being from the ground up.

Creating a Personalized Reflexology Plan

The beauty of reflexology lies in its versatility. Unlike a one-size-fits-all approach, it allows you to create a personalized plan that caters to your unique needs and goals. This guide will equip you with the knowledge to design a reflexology routine that optimizes your well-being.

Step 1: Assess Your Needs and Goals

The foundation of your personalized plan begins with introspection. Consider the following:

- **Overall Health:** Do you have any specific health concerns you'd like to address, such as stress, headaches, or digestive issues?

- **Lifestyle Factors:** Do you experience high levels of stress, get inadequate sleep, or have a demanding physical job? These factors can influence reflexology needs.

- **Desired Outcome:** Are you primarily seeking relaxation, targeting specific areas of concern, or aiming for a more holistic approach?

Step 2: Explore Different Reflexology Techniques

With your needs and goals in mind, delve into the various reflexology techniques available:

- **Foot Reflexology:** This is the most common practice, focusing on applying pressure to specific points on the feet. Refer to the reflexology foot chart in the book to identify zones corresponding to your areas of concern.

- **Hand Reflexology:** Similar to the feet, hands also hold a map of reflex points. This can be a convenient option for self-reflexology throughout the day.

- **Ear Reflexology (Auricular Reflexology):** This technique focuses on pressure points on the outer ear, offering a targeted approach for specific concerns.

Step 3: Design Your Reflexology Routine

Now it's time to create your personalized schedule:

- **Frequency:** Aim for consistency. Consider daily sessions for acute concerns or 2-3 sessions per week for general well-being.

- **Duration:** Start with short sessions (5-10 minutes) and gradually increase as comfort allows.

- **Technique Selection:** Choose the technique(s) that best align with your needs and preferences. You can even combine foot and hand reflexology for a more comprehensive approach.

Step 4: Tailoring Your Sessions

Here's how to personalize your reflexology sessions even further:

- **Focus on Specific Areas:** If you have specific concerns, target the corresponding reflex points during your sessions.

- **Pressure Variation:** Adjust the pressure applied based on your needs. Lighter pressure might be suitable for relaxation, while firmer pressure can be used for targeting specific areas.

- **Relaxation Techniques:** Incorporate calming elements like aromatherapy or soothing music to enhance the overall experience.

Step 5: Monitor Progress and Adapt

The key to a successful plan is to monitor its effectiveness:

- **Track Changes:** Pay attention to how you feel after reflexology sessions. Did your stress levels decrease? Did you experience improved sleep?

- **Adjust as Needed:** If certain techniques don't seem to be working, don't hesitate to adjust your routine or seek guidance from a qualified reflexology practitioner.

Additional Tips for a Personalized Reflexology Plan:

- **Listen to Your Body:** Pay attention to any discomfort during reflexology. If something feels painful, adjust your pressure or technique.

- **Hydration is Key:** Drinking plenty of water before and after your reflexology sessions can help facilitate the release of toxins.

- **Maintain a Healthy Lifestyle:** Reflexology is a valuable tool, but it works best when combined with a healthy diet, regular exercise, and adequate sleep.

Remember: Creating a personalized reflexology plan is an ongoing process. Experiment with different techniques and find what works best for you. As you listen to your body and refine your routine, you'll unlock the full potential of reflexology and experience its profound impact on your well-being.

Part 2:
Mastering the Techniques - Putting Reflexology into Practice

Chapter 3:

The Art of Touch: Essential Techniques for Effective Reflexology Sessions

Preparing Yourself and Your Client for Optimal Results

Reflexology is more than just applying pressure to specific points on the feet or hands. It's an art form, a mindful practice that requires a skilled touch and a comfortable environment to achieve optimal results. This chapter delves into the essential techniques for effective reflexology sessions, focusing on preparing yourself and your client for a truly beneficial experience.

Preparing Yourself: The Foundation for Effective Touch

Before embarking on a reflexology session, whether for yourself or a client, it's crucial to ensure you're in the right frame of mind and body. Here are some key steps:

- **Center Yourself:** Take a few minutes to quiet your mind and focus your energy. Deep breathing exercises or meditation can be helpful in achieving a calm and centered state.

- **Hygiene:** Maintain good hygiene by washing your hands thoroughly before and after each session.

- **Trim Your Nails:** Keep your fingernails short and smooth to prevent any discomfort during the session.

- **Warm Your Hands:** Gently rub your hands together or use warm water to create a gentle warmth that will be more comfortable for your client.

- **Hydration:** Stay well-hydrated. This helps maintain the suppleness of your hands, making it easier to apply pressure effectively.

Creating a Welcoming and Relaxing Environment

The environment plays a crucial role in promoting relaxation and enhancing the effectiveness of your reflexology session. Here's how to create an optimal space:

- **Ambiance:** Dim the lights and create a calming atmosphere. Consider using aromatherapy with relaxing essential oils like lavender or chamomile.

- **Comfortable Temperature:** Maintain a comfortable room temperature that's neither too hot nor too cold.

- **Soothing Sounds:** Play soft, calming music or nature sounds to create a peaceful ambiance.

- **Comfortable Surface:** Ensure your client is positioned comfortably on a massage table or a reclining chair with proper head and neck support.

- **Drapes or Blankets:** Provide drapes or blankets for your client to ensure they feel warm and comfortable throughout the session.

Preparing Your Client for Optimal Results

Effective communication and setting clear expectations are vital for a successful reflexology session. Here's how to prepare your client:

- **Consultation:** Discuss the client's health history, any specific concerns they have, and their desired outcome from the session.

- **Informed Consent:** Obtain informed consent from your client after explaining the potential benefits and contraindications of reflexology.

- **Setting Expectations:** Let your client know what to expect during the session, including the techniques used, the amount of pressure applied, and the typical duration.

- **Open Communication:** Encourage your client to communicate any discomfort they experience during the session so you can adjust your pressure or techniques accordingly.

Essential Techniques for Effective Reflexology Sessions

Beyond preparation, mastering the art of touch is essential for an effective reflexology session. Here are some key techniques to remember:

- **Thumb and Finger Walks:** Use firm but gentle strokes with your thumbs or fingers to "walk" over reflex zones on the feet or hands.

- **Static Pressure:** Apply gentle, sustained pressure to specific reflex points for a few seconds before releasing. Breathe in unison with your client for added relaxation.

- **Circular Motions:** On certain reflex points, use small, gentle circular motions to stimulate the area.

- **Holding Techniques:** For some reflex points, you can hold a gentle pinching motion or use a thumb and finger cradle to apply focused pressure.

Remember: Always prioritize comfort. The pressure should be firm but not painful. If your client experiences any discomfort, adjust your technique or focus on different reflex points.

Beyond Technique: The Importance of Empathy and Intuition

While mastering techniques is crucial, the most effective reflexology sessions go beyond mechanics. Here are some additional elements to consider:

- **Empathy:** Approach your client with empathy and a genuine desire to promote their well-being.

- **Intuition:** Pay attention to subtle cues from your client's body and adjust your technique accordingly.

- **Mind-Body Connection:** Remember that reflexology is a holistic practice. Connecting with your client on a human level can enhance the experience.

Basic Reflexology Techniques: Strokes, Presses, and Holds

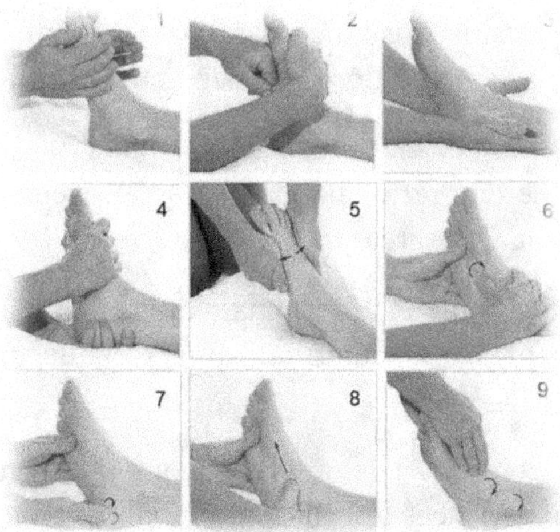

Reflexology relies on the art of touch to stimulate specific reflex points on the feet, hands, or other areas of the body. Mastering these basic techniques – strokes, presses, and holds – will equip you to deliver effective reflexology sessions, promoting relaxation and potentially addressing various concerns.

1. Strokes: Warming Up and Stimulating Reflex Zones

Strokes are gentle movements used to warm up the area, stimulate circulation, and prepare the reflex points for deeper pressure. Here are some common strokes:

- **Thumb Walk:** Gently glide your thumb back and forth across the entire foot or hand, applying light pressure. This helps warm up the area and identify any areas of tenderness.

- **Finger Walk:** Use your index finger or a combination of fingers to walk across reflex zones in a wave-like motion. This helps stimulate specific areas and prepare them for further attention.

- **Feather Strokes:** With a light touch, use your fingertips to brush across reflex zones in short, feathery strokes. This is a gentle way to awaken and stimulate the reflex points.

2. Presses: Applying Focused Pressure to Specific Points

Presses are the core of reflexology, targeting specific reflex points with focused pressure to potentially influence their corresponding organs or systems. Here are some key presses to consider:

- **Static Press:** This is the most basic press. Locate a reflex point and apply firm but gentle pressure with your thumb or finger for 3-5 seconds. Breathe in unison with your client for added relaxation. Release slowly.

- **Circular Press:** On certain reflex points, use a small, gentle circular motion with your thumb or finger for a few seconds. This can be particularly helpful for stimulating congested areas.

- **Thumb and Finger Cradle:** For focused pressure on smaller points, gently cradle the reflex zone between your thumb and finger and apply light to moderate pressure for a few seconds.

3. Holds: Sustained Pressure for Deeper Work

Holds are techniques that involve maintaining pressure on a specific reflex point for a slightly longer duration than a static press. These can be especially helpful for addressing areas of tension or discomfort.

- **Pinching Hold:** Gently pinch the reflex zone between your thumb and finger and hold for 5-7 seconds. This technique can be particularly effective for stimulating congested areas.

- **Thumb Hook:** For some reflex points on the foot, especially on the arch, you can use a "thumb hook" technique. Hook your thumb under the arch and apply gentle but firm pressure upwards for a few seconds.

- **Palm Hold:** This technique applies to larger reflex zones on the hands. Place your palm over the reflex zone and apply gentle, sustained pressure for several seconds.

Important Considerations:

- **Always prioritize comfort:** The pressure applied should be firm but never painful. Adjust your technique based on your client's feedback.

- **Listen to your body:** If you experience discomfort in your hands or wrists while applying pressure, take a break and adjust your body position.

- **Adapt and Experiment:** These are just basic techniques. As you gain experience, experiment with different strokes, presses, and holds to find what works best for you and your client.

Additional Tips for Effective Touch:

- **Maintain a smooth and rhythmic motion:** This creates a calming and focused environment.

- **Use warm hands:** Gently rub your hands together or use warm water to create a gentle warmth for your client.

- **Apply a light lotion or oil (optional):** This can help create smoother hand movements and a more pleasant experience, especially for dry skin.

COMMON CONDITIONS TO TACKLE THROUGH YOUR TOES

SORE THROAT

1. Throat Reflex Point. Start just below the joint of the big toe. 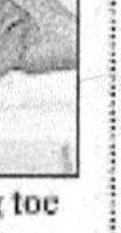 Using your index finger, walk horizontally across the big toe and press into the throat reflex and make circles for seven seconds.

2. Cervical Vertebrae Reflex Area. 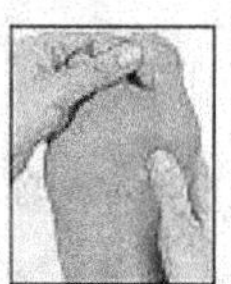 This reflex area lies on the medial aspect of the big toe and in between the joints. Support the big toe with one hand. Use the thumb of the other hand to make seven small steps, remembering that each step represents a specific vertebra. Work towards the foot. Repeat the movement six times.

3. Oesophagus Reflex Area. Flex the foot back with one hand to create skin tension. Place the thumb of your other hand at the diaphragm line in between zones one and two. Work up in between the metatarsals from the diaphragm line to the eye/ear general area. Continue this six times. Working this area can help with disorders of the oesophagus, bad breath and trouble swallowing.

HEARTBURN

1. Diaphragm Reflex Area. 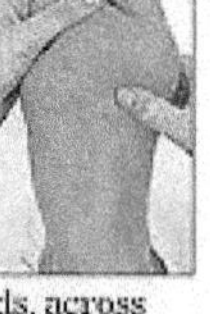 Flex the foot back with one hand to create skin tension. Use the thumb of your other hand to work under the metatarsal heads, across from the lateral aspect to the medial aspect of the foot. Use slow steps and repeat this movement eight times.

2. Oesophagus Reflex Area. 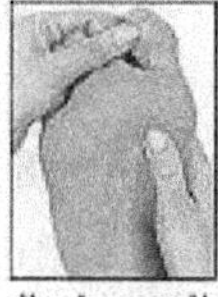 Flex the foot back with one hand to create skin tension. Place the thumb of your other hand at the diaphragm line in between zones one and two. Work up in between the metatarsals from the diaphragm line to the eye/ear general area. Repeat this six times.

3. Pancreas Reflex Point. This reflex point is found only on the right foot. Place your thumb on the third toe and trace a line down to below the diaphragm 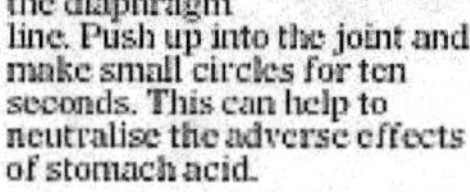 line. Push up into the joint and make small circles for ten seconds. This can help to neutralise the adverse effects of stomach acid.

PREMENSTRUAL SYNDROME (PMS)

1. Pituitary Reflex Point. Support the big toe with the fingers of one hand and use your other thumb to make a cross to find the centre of the big toe. Place 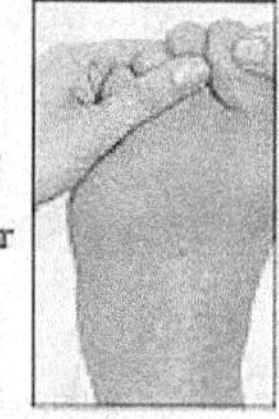 your thumb into the centre, push in and make circles for 15 seconds.

2. Thyroid Reflex Area. 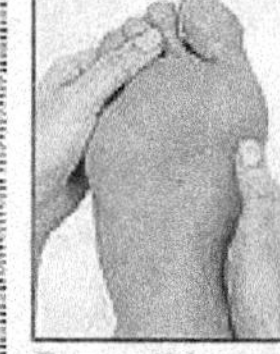 Use the thumb of one hand to work the ball of the foot, from the diaphragm line all the way up to the neckline. Repeat this movement slowly six times over the area.

3. Pancreas Reflex Point. This reflex is found only on the right foot. Use your thumb 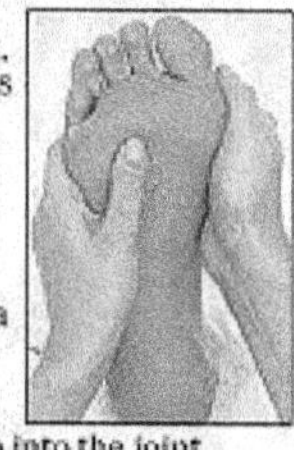 and place it on the third toe, tracing a line down to below the diaphragm line. Push up into the joint, making small circles for 12 seconds.

Advanced Techniques: Tailoring Your Approach for Specific Needs

As you delve deeper into the world of reflexology, you can move beyond basic techniques and explore advanced approaches to tailor your practice to address specific needs. These pages will equip you with valuable insights to personalize reflexology sessions and potentially enhance their effectiveness.

Understanding Reflexology Zones and Corresponding Systems

A foundational understanding of reflexology zone charts (feet, hands, etc.) is crucial for tailoring your approach. These charts map specific points on the feet, hands, ears, or even face to various organs and systems within the body.

- **Consult the Book's Charts:** Refer to the detailed reflexology zone charts included in this book to identify the location of reflex points corresponding to the specific needs you want to target.

- **Research and Explore:** There are many resources available beyond this book that delve deeper into the connections between reflex points and specific body systems.

Tailoring Techniques for Different Needs

Here are some examples of advanced techniques you can incorporate into your sessions to address specific concerns:

- **Relaxation and Stress Relief:**

    - **Focus on Soothing Techniques:** Emphasize gentle strokes, sustained palm holds on the hands, and light circular presses on specific calming reflex points.

- o **Combine with Aromatherapy:** Consider incorporating calming essential oils like lavender or chamomile to enhance the relaxation experience.

- **Headaches and Migraines:**

  - o **Target Reflex Points:** Focus on applying pressure to reflex points associated with the head, neck, and nervous system.

  - o **Sequential Techniques:** Try using sequential strokes or presses, moving from the toes or fingers upwards towards the head to promote a draining effect.

- **Digestive Issues:**

  - o **Reflex Point Focus:** Target reflex points related to the stomach, intestines, and colon. Techniques like gentle kneading or finger walks can be helpful.

  - o **Rhythm and Pressure:** Experiment with applying pressure in a rhythmic pattern that mimics healthy peristalsis (muscular contractions that move food through the digestive system).

Advanced Considerations:

- **Sequencing:** Plan the order in which you address different reflex zones during your session. Consider starting with calming techniques and then progressing to address specific concerns.

- **Refined Pressure:** As you gain experience, you can experiment with more refined pressure variations. For instance, lighter pressure for relaxation and deeper, more focused pressure for specific concerns. Always prioritize comfort.

- **Combination Techniques:** Don't be afraid to combine different strokes, presses, and holds within a single session to create a more dynamic and potentially more effective experience.

Remember: There's no "one size fits all" approach in reflexology. Advanced techniques empower you to personalize your sessions based on your own needs or those of your clients. Listen to your body or your client's feedback and adjust your techniques accordingly.

Exploring Beyond Basic Techniques

The world of reflexology offers a vast array of advanced techniques to explore. Here are some suggestions to consider as you expand your knowledge:

- **Reflexology on the Hands and Ears:** While the feet are the most common focus, reflexology can be practiced on the hands and ears as well. These areas offer additional reflex points that can be targeted for specific needs.

- **Reflexology with Tools:** Some practitioners utilize specialized reflexology tools to apply pressure. These tools can be particularly helpful if you have limitations in hand strength or endurance.

- **Water Reflexology:** This advanced technique involves soaking the feet in warm water infused with essential oils or herbal blends while applying reflexology techniques.

Always consult a qualified reflexology professional before attempting any advanced techniques, especially if you have any underlying health conditions.

Chapter 4:

Beyond Reflexology: Complementary Techniques to Enhance Your Practice

Aroma Reflexology: The Power of Essential Oils

This chapter explores the art of Aroma Reflexology, a practice that combines the benefits of reflexology with the therapeutic properties of essential oils, creating a truly multi-sensory experience. However, the world of holistic well-being extends beyond reflexology.

The Power of Essential Oils

Essential oils are concentrated liquids extracted from various plant parts like flowers, leaves, or seeds. They possess a vast array of therapeutic properties, influencing our mood, promoting relaxation, and even offering potential pain relief. By incorporating essential oils into your reflexology practice, you can enhance the overall experience and potentially amplify the benefits for your client.

Aromatherapy and Reflexology: A Perfect Blend

The sense of smell plays a powerful role in our emotional and physical well-being. When combined with reflexology, essential oils can create a synergistic effect, promoting deeper relaxation and potentially addressing specific concerns more effectively. Here's how Aroma Reflexology works:

- **Olfactory Stimulation:** As you diffuse or apply essential oils during a reflexology session, the pleasant aromas are inhaled and stimulate the olfactory system. This can trigger emotional responses like relaxation or improved mood.

- **Topical Absorption:** Essential oils applied topically on the feet or hands during reflexology can be absorbed through the skin, potentially influencing the body on a cellular level.

Choosing Essential Oils for Reflexology

With a plethora of essential oils available, selecting the right ones for your client can feel overwhelming. Here are some key considerations:

- **Client's Needs:** Consider your client's specific goals. Do they seek relaxation, pain relief, or improved sleep? Choose essential oils known for their properties that complement these needs.

- **Aromatherapy Knowledge:** Familiarize yourself with the therapeutic properties of different essential oils. Consult reputable aromatherapy resources for detailed information.

- **Safety First:** Always prioritize safety. Some essential oils can be irritating or pose health risks for certain individuals. Dilute them properly using a carrier oil like almond or jojoba oil before application.

Here are some popular essential oils for Aroma Reflexology and their potential benefits:

- **Lavender:** Promotes relaxation and reduces anxiety.

- **Peppermint:** Stimulates circulation and may alleviate headaches.

- **Chamomile:** Calms the nervous system and promotes sleep.

- **Roman Chamomile:** Soothes inflammation and promotes relaxation.

- **Sandalwood:** Grounding and calming, may ease anxiety and improve mood.

Important Considerations:

- **Patch Test:** Before applying any essential oil on your client, perform a patch test on a small area of their skin to check for any allergic reactions.

- **Pregnancy and Medical Conditions:** Certain essential oils are contraindicated for pregnant or breastfeeding women and individuals with specific medical conditions. Always consult with the client's doctor before using essential oils.

- **Less is More:** A few drops of essential oil diluted in a carrier oil is sufficient. Avoid overusing essential oils to prevent irritation.

Enhancing Your Reflexology Practice with Aroma Reflexology

- **Diffuse Essential Oils:** Create a calming atmosphere by diffusing a blend of essential oils suitable for your client's needs during the session.

- **Apply Diluted Essential Oils:** After consulting with your client and ensuring safety, apply diluted essential oils directly to specific reflex points on the feet or hands. Gently massage the oil into the area, combining the pressure of reflexology with the benefits of aromatherapy.

- **Create a Customized Blend:** Explore creating custom essential oil blends based on your client's specific needs and preferences. This adds a personalized touch to your Aroma Reflexology practice.

Remember: Aroma Reflexology is a powerful tool to elevate your reflexology practice and potentially provide an even more profound and enjoyable experience for your clients.

Warm Stone Therapy: Adding a Touch of Soothing Warmth

This section delves into Warm Stone Therapy, a technique that utilizes heated stones to create a deeply relaxing and potentially therapeutic experience when combined with reflexology.

The Benefits of Warm Stone Therapy

Warm stones offer a unique sensory experience that complements reflexology in several ways:

- **Muscle Relaxation:** The heat from the stones helps to relax tense muscles, making them more receptive to the pressure applied during reflexology.

- **Improved Circulation:** The warmth can promote blood flow throughout the body, potentially aiding in the removal of toxins and enhancing the overall effectiveness of reflexology.

- **Enhanced Relaxation:** The warmth from the stones can be deeply comforting and promote a sense of peace and relaxation, further amplifying the benefits of reflexology.

What You'll Need for Warm Stone Therapy

To incorporate warm stone therapy into your reflexology practice, you'll need a few essential items:

- **Basalt Stones:** These smooth, volcanic stones are ideal for retaining heat. Choose a variety of sizes to target different reflex points on the feet or hands.

- **Stone Heater:** Invest in a specifically designed stone heater to safely and consistently warm the stones to a comfortable temperature (around 130-145 degrees Fahrenheit).

- **Towels:** Have a few clean towels on hand to use for drying the stones and for client comfort.

- **Carrier Oil (Optional):** A light carrier oil like almond or jojoba oil can help the stones glide smoothly over the skin and enhance the experience.

Steps for Incorporating Warm Stone Therapy into Reflexology

Here's a step-by-step guide to integrating warm stones into your reflexology sessions:

1. **Preparation:** Heat the stones in the stone heater to the desired temperature (consult your heater's instructions). While the stones are warming up, prepare the reflexology environment and ensure your client is comfortable.

2. **Stone Placement:** Once the stones are warm, carefully remove them from the heater using a towel or tongs. Begin your reflexology session using your usual techniques. As you work on specific reflex points, strategically place warm stones on those areas.

3. **Stone Application:** You can hold the stones in place on specific reflex points or use them to gently glide over reflex zones in combination with your reflexology techniques. The warmth from the stones will enhance the pressure and potentially deepen the relaxation response.

4. **Temperature Monitoring:** Throughout the session, periodically check the temperature of the stones to ensure they remain comfortable for your client. You can also offer the client a cool towel to periodically place on their forehead if needed.

5. **Stone Removal:** As you complete your reflexology routine, gently remove the stones. Allow your client time to relax and enjoy the lingering warmth before ending the session.

Important Considerations:

- **Client Comfort:** Always prioritize client comfort. The stones should be warm, not hot. Adjust the temperature or remove stones if your client feels any discomfort.

- **Communication:** Communicate clearly with your client throughout the session. Ask them about their comfort level and adjust your technique or stone placement accordingly.

- **Contraindications:** Warm stone therapy may not be suitable for everyone. Be aware of contraindications such as pregnancy, fever, or certain skin conditions. Consult with your client's doctor if unsure.

Adding Warm Stone Therapy to Your Reflexology Practice

Incorporating warm stone therapy into your reflexology sessions, you can create a truly luxurious and potentially more therapeutic experience for your clients. The combination of reflexology techniques with the soothing warmth of the stones can promote deeper relaxation, enhance circulation, and potentially address muscle tension more effectively. Remember, prioritize client comfort, maintain clear communication, and be mindful of any contraindications to ensure a safe and beneficial experience.

Integrating Reflexology with Other Relaxation Techniques

These pages explore how reflexology can be harmoniously blended with other modalities to create a symphony of relaxation and well-being:

1. Guided Meditation and Mindfulness:

- **The Synergy:** Combine reflexology with guided meditation to create a deeply relaxing and introspective experience. While you apply reflexology techniques, guide your client through calming imagery or breathing exercises. This can enhance the focus and potentially amplify the stress-reducing benefits of both practices.

- **How to Integrate:** Begin your session with a short-guided meditation to help your client center themselves. Intersperse periods of reflexology with brief mindfulness prompts, encouraging your client to focus on their breath and bodily sensations. End the session with a guided meditation to solidify the relaxation response.

2. Deep Breathing Techniques:

- **The Synergy:** Incorporating deep breathing exercises into your reflexology sessions can significantly enhance the relaxation experience. Focused breathing patterns can activate the parasympathetic nervous system, promoting relaxation and potentially lowering blood pressure.

- **How to Integrate:** Before or during your reflexology routine, guide your client through a few cycles of deep belly breathing. Inhale slowly through the nose, allowing the belly to expand, and exhale completely through the mouth. Synchronize the breath with your reflexology techniques for added focus.

3. Aromatherapy with Essential Oils (Beyond Aroma Reflexology):

- **The Synergy:** While Aroma Reflexology combines essential oils directly with reflexology, this section explores using essential oils in a complementary way. Diffusing essential oils with calming properties can create a relaxing atmosphere and enhance the overall experience.

- **How to Integrate:** Choose essential oils known for their relaxing or stress-reducing properties like lavender, chamomile, or sandalwood. Diffuse them throughout the session to create a calming ambiance that complements the reflexology techniques.

4. Soothing Music Therapy:

- **The Synergy:** Carefully selected music can have a profound impact on mood and relaxation. Incorporating calming music into your reflexology session can set the tone for a peaceful experience and potentially enhance the therapeutic effects.

- **How to Integrate:** Create a playlist with calming instrumental music, nature sounds, or binaural beats. Adjust the volume to ensure it's subtle and doesn't overpower the session. The music should create a peaceful backdrop rather than a distraction.

5. Visualization Techniques:

- **The Synergy:** Visualization techniques can be a powerful tool for promoting relaxation and enhancing self-healing. By guiding your client through positive imagery, you can help them focus on a sense of calm and well-being, complementing the benefits of reflexology.

- **How to Integrate:** After applying reflexology techniques to specific areas, introduce calming visualizations that correspond to those areas. For example, focusing on the reflex points for the head, guide your client to visualize a peaceful scene or a sense of clarity.

Remember:

- **Tailor the Experience:** The key to successful integration lies in understanding your client's needs and preferences. Ask them what relaxation techniques they enjoy and choose modalities that complement their goals.

- **Create a Seamless Flow:** The integration should feel natural and flow smoothly within the reflexology session. Experiment with different combinations to find what works best for you and your clients.

- **Safety First:** Be aware of any contraindications for the chosen relaxation techniques. Always prioritize the safety and well-being of your client.

Part 3:
Unlocking the Benefits - Reflexology's Impact on Your Wellbeing

Chapter 5:

Stress Less, Live More: How Reflexology Can Help Manage Stress and Anxiety

Understanding the Stress Response and its Impact on Health

The modern world throws a constant barrage of stressors our way, from work deadlines to traffic jams and everything in between. This chronic stress can wreak havoc on our physical and emotional well-being, leaving us feeling frazzled, anxious, and depleted. But there's hope! Reflexology, the practice of applying pressure to specific points on the feet or hands, offers a natural and non-invasive approach to managing stress and anxiety, helping you reclaim your inner calm and live a more vibrant life.

Understanding the Stress Response and its Impact on Health

Before diving into how reflexology combats stress, let's explore the body's natural stress response, often referred to as "fight-or-flight." When faced with a perceived threat, our bodies release a surge of hormones like adrenaline and cortisol. This prepares us to either confront the threat or flee the situation. While this response is crucial for survival in the short term, chronic stress keeps our bodies in a constant state of fight-or-flight, leading to a cascade of negative health consequences:

- **Weakened Immune System:** Chronic stress can suppress the immune system, making us more susceptible to illness.

- **Digestive Issues:** Stress can disrupt digestion, leading to constipation, diarrhea, or even stomach ulcers.

- **Muscle Tension and Headaches:** Stress often manifests as physical tension in the muscles, particularly in the neck and shoulders, and can contribute to headaches.

- **Anxiety and Sleep Problems:** Chronic stress can fuel anxiety and make it difficult to fall asleep or stay asleep, creating a vicious cycle.

How Reflexology Can Help Break the Stress Cycle

Reflexology offers a multifaceted approach to combating stress and its associated concerns. Here's how:

- **Promotes Relaxation:** By stimulating specific reflex points, reflexology can trigger the release of feel-good chemicals like endorphins, which naturally promote relaxation and reduce stress hormones like cortisol.

- **Improves Blood Circulation:** Reflexology techniques can enhance blood flow throughout the body, which helps to reduce muscle tension and promotes a sense of calm.

- **Boosts the Nervous System:** Reflexology can stimulate the parasympathetic nervous system, which is responsible for our relaxation response. This helps to counter the effects of the fight-or-flight response and promotes feelings of peace and well-being.

- **Improves Sleep Quality:** By promoting relaxation and reducing anxiety, reflexology can help pave the way for better sleep, a crucial element in stress management.

Integrating Reflexology into Your Stress Management Routine

Here are some tips for incorporating reflexology into your stress management routine:

- **Schedule Regular Sessions:** Aim for 2-3 reflexology sessions per week, or even daily short sessions, to experience the cumulative benefits in managing stress.

- **Create a Relaxing Environment:** Dim the lights, light some calming candles, or play soothing music to enhance the relaxation response during your self-reflexology sessions or when visiting a reflexologist.

- **Combine with Other Stress-Reduction Techniques:** Reflexology is a powerful tool, but it's most effective when combined with other stress-management techniques like exercise, meditation, or deep breathing exercises.

- **Listen to Your Body:** Pay attention to how your body responds to reflexology. If you experience any discomfort, adjust the pressure or focus on different reflex points.

Remember: Stress management is a journey, not a destination. By incorporating reflexology into your life, you'll equip yourself with a powerful tool to combat stress, promote relaxation, and cultivate a sense of well-being that allows you to truly stress less and live more.

Reflexology's Role in Promoting Relaxation and Reducing Tension

In today's fast-paced world, our bodies often hold onto tension like a clenched fist. This chronic tension can manifest in various ways, from tight muscles and headaches to difficulty sleeping and a general sense of unease. Fortunately, reflexology offers a natural and gentle approach to promoting relaxation and reducing tension, helping you unwind and rediscover inner peace.

Understanding the Tension-Relaxation Cycle

Our bodies have a built-in tension-relaxation cycle. When faced with stress or physical exertion, muscles naturally tense up to protect us and provide stability. However, when this tension isn't released through movement or relaxation techniques, it can become chronic, leading to discomfort and a state of dis-ease.

Reflexology: A Gateway to Relaxation

Reflexology works by stimulating specific reflex points on the feet or hands, believed to correspond with various organs and systems within the body. This targeted pressure can trigger a cascade of beneficial responses that promote relaxation and reduce tension:

- **Stimulates the Nervous System:** By activating the parasympathetic nervous system, reflexology encourages the body to shift from its "fight-or-flight" stress response to a relaxed state. This can lead to a decrease in heart rate, muscle tension, and overall feelings of anxiety.

- **Promotes the Release of Endorphins:** Reflexology techniques can stimulate the release of endorphins, the body's natural painkillers and mood elevators. This creates a sense of well-being and reduces the perception of pain associated with tension headaches or muscle stiffness.

- **Improves Blood Circulation:** Reflexology techniques like strokes and presses can enhance blood flow throughout the body. This increased circulation helps deliver oxygen and nutrients to the muscles, promoting relaxation and aiding in the removal of waste products that contribute to tension.

Techniques for Fostering Relaxation During Reflexology

There are specific reflexology techniques that can be particularly helpful in promoting relaxation and reducing tension:

- **Feather Strokes:** These gentle, brushing motions across reflex zones warm up the area and create a calming sensation.

- **Static Presses:** Applying firm but gentle pressure to specific reflex points for a few seconds can help release deep-seated tension and promote a sense of groundedness.

- **Circular Motions:** Using small, gentle circles on specific reflex points can stimulate circulation and encourage a feeling of release.

Beyond Technique: Creating a Relaxing Environment

For optimal relaxation during a reflexology session, consider incorporating the following elements:

- **Dim Lighting:** Soft lighting creates a calming ambiance and encourages the body to unwind.

- **Soothing Aromatherapy:** Essential oils like lavender or chamomile can evoke feelings of peace and tranquility.

- **Serene Music:** Soft, calming music can further enhance the relaxation response and promote a sense of well-being.

Reflexology: A Journey Towards Inner Peace

Reflexology is more than just a technique; it's a journey toward inner peace. By incorporating regular reflexology sessions into your life, you can combat the negative effects of tension, promote relaxation, and cultivate a sense of calm that permeates all aspects of your well-being. Remember, consistent practice is key. As you continue your reflexology journey, you'll discover its profound ability to melt away tension, leaving you feeling centered, relaxed, and ready to embrace a more peaceful state of being.

Enhancing Sleep Quality Through Reflexology Techniques

For many, a good night's sleep feels like a distant dream. Tossing and turning, battling racing thoughts, and waking up feeling unrested can significantly impact our daily lives. Fortunately, reflexology offers a natural and drug-free approach to promoting better sleep, helping you drift off more easily and wake feeling refreshed.

Understanding the Sleep Cycle and its Disruptions

Sleep is a complex biological process vital for physical and mental rejuvenation. We cycle through various stages of sleep throughout the night, each playing a crucial role in our health and well-being. However, various factors can disrupt this delicate cycle, leading to sleep disturbances:

- **Stress and Anxiety:** Worrying thoughts and a hyperactive mind can make it difficult to quiet down and fall asleep.

- **Muscle Tension:** Tight muscles throughout the body can create physical discomfort that hinders relaxation and sleep initiation.

- **Hormonal Imbalances:** Fluctuations in hormones like melatonin, responsible for regulating our sleep-wake cycle, can contribute to insomnia.

Reflexology: A Pathway to a Restful Night

Reflexology can address various sleep disruptors by influencing the body's natural sleep-promoting mechanisms:

- **Promotes Relaxation:** By stimulating specific reflex points, reflexology can activate the parasympathetic nervous system, encouraging the body to shift into a relaxed state. This decrease in stress hormones like cortisol helps create an environment conducive to sleep.

- **Reduces Muscle Tension:** Reflexology techniques can help release tightness and discomfort in the muscles, creating a more relaxed physical state that promotes restful sleep.

- **Improves Blood Circulation:** Enhanced blood flow, facilitated by reflexology techniques, promotes the delivery of oxygen and nutrients to the body, which is crucial for relaxation and sleep.

- **Boosts the Nervous System:** Reflexology can stimulate the production of neurotransmitters like serotonin, which plays a role in regulating sleep patterns and promoting feelings of well-being.

Reflexology Techniques for a Better Night's Sleep

Here are some reflexology techniques you can utilize to promote sleep:

- **Solar Plexus Reflex:** Locate the solar plexus reflex on the sole of the foot, just below the diaphragm. Apply gentle, circular motions with your thumb for a few seconds. This point is believed to influence the nervous system and promote relaxation.

- **Spleen Reflex:** Find the spleen reflex on the inner arch of the foot. Apply a static press with your thumb for a few seconds. This reflex point is believed to correspond with energy levels and can be helpful for individuals struggling with anxiety-related sleep disturbances.

- **Brain Reflex:** Situated on the big toe, the brain reflex is believed to influence the nervous system and promote calmness. Gently massage this area using strokes or light circular motions.

Creating a Sleep-Promoting Environment with Reflexology

Beyond specific techniques, creating a sleep-conducive environment plays a crucial role in reflexology for sleep:

- **Nighttime Routine:** Schedule regular reflexology sessions before bed to establish a relaxing bedtime ritual.

- **Dim Lighting:** Dim the lights in the room to signal to your body that it's time to wind down.

- **Calming Aromatherapy:** Diffuse essential oils like lavender or chamomile during your reflexology session to create a tranquil atmosphere.

Reflexology: A Gentle Journey Towards Better Sleep

Reflexology isn't a magic bullet for sleep, but it offers a gentle and natural approach to promoting better sleep hygiene. By incorporating regular reflexology sessions into your nighttime routine and creating a sleep-supportive environment, you can unlock its potential to lull yourself into a deeper, more restful sleep. Remember, consistency is key. As you integrate reflexology into your sleep routine, you might discover a significant improvement in your sleep quality, leaving you feeling more refreshed and energized throughout the day.

Chapter 6:

A Journey Towards Wholeness: The Benefits of Reflexology for Overall Health

Boosting the Immune System and Promoting Detoxification

The human body is a magnificent machine, constantly working to maintain optimal health. But sometimes, amidst the daily hustle and environmental challenges, our well-being can falter. This is where reflexology steps in, offering a holistic approach that supports the body's natural ability to heal and thrive. This chapter delves into how reflexology can bolster the immune system and promote detoxification, paving the way for a more balanced and resilient state of health.

Understanding the Pillars of Wholeness: Immunity and Detoxification

- **The Mighty Immune System:** Our immune system acts as a vigilant defender, constantly on guard against invading pathogens like bacteria and viruses. A strong immune system is crucial for fighting off illness and maintaining overall health.

- **The Detoxification Dance:** Our bodies are constantly accumulating waste products from everyday cellular processes and environmental exposure. Detoxification is the body's natural way of eliminating these unwanted elements, promoting optimal function.

Reflexology: A Supportive Ally

While reflexology isn't a replacement for conventional medicine, it offers a complementary approach that can support the body's natural defense mechanisms and detoxification processes:

- **Boosting the Immune System:** Reflexology may influence the immune system by stimulating specific reflex points believed to correspond to the thymus gland and lymphatic system. The thymus plays a vital role in the development of white blood cells, the body's soldiers in the fight against infection. The lymphatic system acts as a waste disposal network, flushing out toxins and cellular debris. By stimulating these reflex points, reflexology may help to enhance the overall function of the immune system.

- **Promoting Detoxification:** Reflexology techniques that promote circulation, such as gentle strokes and kneading, may encourage the body to more effectively eliminate waste products through the lymphatic system, kidneys, and skin. This can help reduce the burden on the body and support overall well-being.

Reflexology Techniques to Enhance Wholeness

Here are some reflexology techniques you can utilize to potentially support your immune system and detoxification:

- **Thymus Reflex:** Locate the thymus reflex on the upper chest of the foot, just below the big toe joint. Apply gentle circular motions with your thumb for a few seconds on each foot.

- **Lymphatic Drainage Techniques:** Utilize gentle strokes moving upwards from the toes towards the ankle and up the leg. This may encourage the flow of lymph fluid, promoting the removal of waste products.

- **Reflex Points for Elimination Organs:** Focus on reflex points corresponding to the kidneys, liver, and intestines. These organs play a crucial role in detoxification. Utilize gentle static presses or stroking techniques on these reflex points.

Enhancing the Benefits of Reflexology

To maximize the potential benefits of reflexology for boosting immunity and promoting detoxification, consider these additional tips:

- **Hydration is Key:** Drinking plenty of water throughout the day facilitates detoxification and helps the body eliminate waste products.

- **Healthy Diet:** Fuel your body with nutritious foods rich in vitamins, minerals, and antioxidants to support immune function.

- **Manage Stress:** Chronic stress can weaken the immune system. Practice stress-reduction techniques like meditation or deep breathing alongside reflexology.

Reflexology is a journey towards a more balanced and resilient you. By incorporating regular reflexology sessions into your life, you can potentially support your immune system, promote detoxification, and contribute to a sense of overall well-being

Improving Circulation and Pain Management

Our bodies are intricate networks of interconnected systems. One crucial system, the circulatory system, acts like a complex river network, delivering oxygen and nutrients to every cell while removing waste products. When circulation falters, it can lead to a cascade of issues, including pain, fatigue, and even tissue damage. Fortunately, reflexology offers a natural and non-invasive approach to potentially improve circulation and offer relief from pain.

Understanding Circulation and its Impact

- **The Flow of Life:** Blood circulation is the body's internal delivery system. It carries oxygen, nutrients, and hormones throughout the body, while simultaneously removing waste products like carbon dioxide.

- **The Ripple Effect of Poor Circulation:** When circulation becomes sluggish, tissues don't receive the oxygen and nutrients they need to function optimally. This can lead to pain, fatigue, numbness, and even difficulty healing from injuries.

Reflexology: A Boost for Circulation

Reflexology techniques can potentially improve circulation by influencing various physiological pathways:

- **Stimulating the Nervous System:** By activating the parasympathetic nervous system, reflexology can encourage relaxation and potentially lower blood pressure. This relaxed state allows blood vessels to dilate, improving blood flow throughout the body.

- **Enhancing Lymphatic Drainage:** The lymphatic system acts as a secondary circulatory system, transporting waste products and excess fluid away from tissues. Reflexology techniques that promote lymphatic drainage, like gentle strokes towards the heart, may help eliminate these waste products and improve overall circulation.

- **Muscle Relaxation:** Tight muscles can impede blood flow. Reflexology techniques that address muscle tension may indirectly improve circulation by allowing blood to flow more freely through relaxed tissues.

Reflexology Techniques for Improved Circulation and Pain Management

Here are some reflexology techniques you can utilize to potentially improve circulation and manage pain:

- **Foot Reflex for the Arch:** Locate the arch reflex on the sole of the foot. Utilize gentle stroking motions from the heel towards the toes to stimulate circulation in the feet.

- **Solar Plexus Reflex:** Situated on the sole of the foot, just below the diaphragm, lies the solar plexus reflex. Apply gentle, circular motions with your thumb for a few seconds. This point may influence the nervous system and promote relaxation, potentially reducing pain associated with tension.

- **Reflex Points for Specific Ailments:** For targeted pain management, consult a reflexology chart to identify reflex points corresponding to specific areas of discomfort (e.g., headaches, back pain). Apply gentle pressure or stroking techniques on these points.

Enhancing the Benefits of Reflexology

To maximize the potential benefits of reflexology for circulation and pain management, consider these additional tips:

- **Hydration is Key:** Drinking plenty of water helps to thin the blood and facilitates better circulation.

- **Healthy Diet:** A diet rich in fruits, vegetables, and whole grains provides essential nutrients that support healthy blood vessels and circulation.

- **Regular Exercise:** Regular physical activity promotes healthy blood flow and can help manage pain through the release of endorphins.

Supporting Specific Health Conditions (e.g., headaches, digestive issues)

Life throws various curveballs, and sometimes these manifest as physical discomfort. Common ailments like headaches and digestive issues can disrupt our daily routines and leave us feeling drained. While reflexology isn't a replacement for medical diagnosis or treatment, it can offer a complementary approach to support specific health conditions and potentially promote a sense of relief and well-being.

Understanding Your Discomfort: Headaches and Digestive Issues

- **The Throbbing Torment of Headaches:** Headaches can have various causes, ranging from stress and tension to dehydration and underlying medical conditions.

- **The Rumbling Discomfort of Digestive Issues:** Digestive issues like constipation, bloating, and heartburn can be caused by dietary choices, stress, or even gut imbalances.

Reflexology: A Targeted Ally

Reflexology can potentially address specific health conditions by focusing on reflex points believed to correspond with different bodily systems:

- **Headache Relief:** Reflexology techniques that promote relaxation, such as gentle strokes on the solar plexus reflex (located on the sole of the foot, just below the diaphragm), may help reduce tension headaches. Additionally, applying pressure to specific head reflex points on the toes or the instep might provide targeted relief.

- **Digestive Support:** Reflexology techniques that stimulate the digestive system can be helpful. Applying gentle pressure or strokes on reflex points corresponding to the stomach, intestines, and colon may encourage digestive motility and potentially alleviate symptoms like constipation and bloating.

Important Considerations:

- **While reflexology can offer relief for some individuals, it's crucial to consult a healthcare professional for persistent or severe headaches or digestive issues.** Early diagnosis and appropriate treatment are essential for managing these conditions effectively.

- **Reflexology techniques for specific health conditions should be tailored to the individual's needs.** Severity, cause, and overall health status will influence the type and intensity of pressure applied to specific reflex points.

A Guide to Reflexology Techniques for Specific Conditions

Headaches:

- **Solar Plexus Reflex:** As mentioned earlier, stimulating this reflex point can promote relaxation and potentially alleviate tension headaches.

- **Head Reflex Points:** Locate reflex points on the big toe (forehead), second toe (eyes), and third toe (sinuses) according to a reflexology chart. Apply gentle pressure or strokes for a few seconds on each point.

Digestive Issues:

- **Stomach Reflex:** Situated on the ball of the foot, the stomach reflex can be stimulated with gentle circular motions to potentially enhance digestive function.

- **Intestine Reflexes:** Locate the small and large intestine reflexes on the sole of the foot, typically running along the outer and inner edges. Utilize gentle strokes or kneading techniques to encourage intestinal motility.

- **Colon Reflex:** Found on the descending arch of the foot, the colon reflex can be stimulated with gentle strokes moving upwards towards the ankle. This may help promote elimination and alleviate constipation.

Remember:

Consistency is key. Regular reflexology sessions, combined with a healthy lifestyle and appropriate medical care when needed, can potentially support the management of specific health conditions and contribute to a sense of overall well-being. As you embark on this journey, you might discover a natural approach to finding relief and promoting a healthier, happier you.

Part 4:
Reflexology for Everyone? Safety Considerations and Special Cases

Chapter 7:

Creating a Safe and Effective Reflexology Practice

Contraindications and Conditions Where Reflexology Should be Avoided

Reflexology offers a wealth of potential benefits, but like any health practice, it's crucial to approach it with safety and awareness. This chapter delves into contraindications, situations where reflexology should be avoided, ensuring you create a safe and effective reflexology practice for yourself or others.

Understanding Contraindications: When Reflexology Might Not Be Your Best Choice

There are certain circumstances where reflexology may not be suitable, and seeking medical advice is essential before proceeding. Here are some key contraindications to be aware of:

- **Acute Injuries:** Reflexology is not recommended on areas with recent fractures, sprains, or injuries. Applying pressure on these areas can worsen inflammation and impede healing.

- **Infections:** Avoid reflexology if you have an active infection, such as a fever, cold, or flu. Reflexology might stimulate the lymphatic system, potentially spreading the infection further.

- **Thrombosis or Blood Clots:** Individuals with a history of blood clots or at risk of developing them should avoid reflexology, as stimulating circulation could dislodge a clot and lead to serious complications.

- **High-Risk Pregnancies:** Reflexology is generally not recommended during the first trimester of pregnancy due to the risk of stimulating uterine contractions. Consult a healthcare professional and a qualified prenatal reflexologist if considering reflexology during later stages of pregnancy.

- **Certain Medical Conditions:** If you have any pre-existing medical conditions, such as heart disease, epilepsy, or uncontrolled diabetes, consult your doctor before receiving reflexology. They can advise you on whether it's a safe and suitable practice for you.

Creating a Safe and Respectful Environment

Here are some additional tips for a safe and effective reflexology practice:

- **Open Communication:** Maintain open communication with the person receiving reflexology. Ask about any pain or discomfort they experience and adjust pressure accordingly.

- **Hygiene is Key:** Maintain good hygiene by washing hands thoroughly before and after a reflexology session. Use clean towels and linens.

- **Respect Individual Preferences:** Not everyone enjoys the same level of pressure. Start with gentle pressure and increase gradually as tolerated. Be mindful of sensitive areas on the feet.

- **Seek Qualified Guidance:** If you're new to reflexology, consider seeking guidance from a qualified reflexologist. They can tailor a session to your specific needs and ensure proper technique.

Remember:

Reflexology is a complementary therapy, not a replacement for medical diagnosis or treatment. If you have any concerns about your health, always consult a qualified healthcare professional.

Maintaining Professional Ethics and Client Communication

The human foot holds a map to our well-being, and as a reflexologist, you have the privilege of guiding clients on a journey of self-discovery and potential healing through reflexology. But this journey requires trust, established through ethical conduct and open communication. These pages explores the importance of maintaining professional ethics and fostering clear communication with your clients.

The Cornerstone of Trust: Ethical Conduct

Reflexology is a powerful tool, and with its use comes a responsibility to adhere to ethical principles. Here are some key aspects of professional ethics for reflexologists:

- **Client Confidentiality:** All information shared by clients during a session, including their medical history and any personal details, must be kept confidential. Maintain detailed client records securely and only share this information with their consent or as required by law.

- **Honesty and Transparency:** Be honest about the limitations of reflexology. It's a complementary therapy, not a substitute for medical diagnosis or treatment. Manage client expectations by explaining that reflexology can support well-being but doesn't guarantee specific results.

- **Informed Consent:** Obtain informed consent from each client before commencing a reflexology session. Explain the techniques used, potential benefits and risks, and answer any questions they may have.

- **Respectful Boundaries:** Maintain professional boundaries with your clients. Avoid self-promotion or offering medical advice beyond your scope of practice.

- **Continuing Education:** Demonstrate your commitment to continuous learning by attending workshops and staying updated on the latest advancements in reflexology research and best practices.

Building Rapport Through Effective Communication

Clear and open communication is vital for building trust and rapport with your clients. Here are some tips for effective communication:

- **Active Listening:** Actively listen to your clients' concerns and goals. Ask open-ended questions to understand their unique needs and expectations.

- **Clear and Concise Explanations:** Explain reflexology techniques and potential benefits in clear and understandable language. Avoid technical jargon and tailor your explanations to the client's level of understanding.

- **Empathy and Compassion:** Approach your clients with empathy and compassion. Acknowledge their concerns and celebrate their progress along the way.

- **Two-Way Communication:** Encourage clients to communicate openly throughout the session. Ask them about their comfort level and adjust pressure or techniques accordingly.

- **Maintaining Professionalism:** Maintain a professional demeanor throughout your interactions with clients. Dress appropriately and project a calm and confident presence.

The Importance of Self-Care for the Reflexology Practitioner

The world of reflexology revolves around the well-being of others. As a reflexologist, your hands become conduits for promoting relaxation, managing pain, and fostering a sense of holistic health. But just like the clients you guide, you too require self-care to maintain your own well-being and ensure you can continue offering your healing touch. These pages delves into the importance of self-care for reflexology practitioners, providing strategies to nurture the healer within.

The Unspoken Risk: Compassion Fatigue and Burnout

Continuously holding space for others' challenges and emotions can take its toll. Reflexology practitioners are susceptible to compassion fatigue, a state of emotional and physical exhaustion brought on by prolonged exposure to the suffering of others. Burnout, characterized by cynicism, emotional detachment, and a sense of ineffectiveness, can also creep in. By prioritizing self-care, you safeguard yourself from these risks and maintain the energy and empathy essential for your practice.

Building a Self-Care Sanctuary

Self-care isn't a luxury; it's a necessity. Here are some strategies to build a self-care sanctuary and nurture the healer within:

- **Maintaining Physical Health:** Prioritize your physical well-being. Eat a nutritious diet, get regular exercise, and ensure adequate sleep. A healthy body fuels a vibrant and resilient spirit.

- **Mindfulness Practices:** Integrate mindfulness practices like meditation or deep breathing into your daily routine. These practices help manage stress, improve focus, and cultivate inner peace, all of which are crucial for effective self-care.

- **Setting Boundaries:** Establish clear boundaries between your professional and personal life. Disconnect from work outside of designated hours and schedule time for activities that bring you joy and relaxation.

- **Self-Reflexology:** Don't neglect your own well-being! Schedule regular self-reflexology sessions to manage stress, promote relaxation, and address any aches or pains you might be experiencing.

- **Supportive Network:** Build a supportive network of friends, family, or colleagues. Having a safe space to share your experiences and challenges can be invaluable for maintaining emotional well-being.

Beyond the Basics: Nurturing Your Passion

Self-care goes beyond just physical and emotional well-being. Nurturing your passion for reflexology is also crucial:

- **Continuing Education:** Stay engaged in your field by attending workshops, conferences, or online courses to expand your knowledge and refine your techniques.

- **Community Connection:** Connect with other reflexology practitioners. Sharing experiences, ideas, and challenges can be a source of inspiration and support.

- **Volunteer Opportunities:** Consider volunteering your skills to offer reflexology to those in need. Giving back to the community can be a deeply rewarding experience that fuels your passion for the practice.

Remember:

You cannot pour from an empty cup. Prioritizing self-care allows you to show up for your clients as your best, most centered self. By nurturing the healer within, you ensure your practice thrives and your passion for reflexology continues to blossom.

Chapter 8:

Reflexology for Special Populations

Adapting Reflexology for Children (Baby Reflexology Techniques)

The world of reflexology isn't limited to adults. This gentle therapy can be surprisingly beneficial for children as well. From soothing a fussy newborn to calming anxiety in a school-aged child, reflexology offers a safe and natural approach to promoting well-being in our little ones. However, their delicate bodies require a specialized approach. This chapter explores adapting reflexology techniques for children, focusing specifically on baby reflexology.

Understanding the Uniqueness of Children:

Children are not simply miniature adults. Their bodies are still developing, and their nervous systems are more sensitive. This necessitates a gentler touch and shorter sessions compared to adult reflexology.

The Power of Touch for Babies:

Touch is one of the most important senses for a newborn baby. It provides comfort, security, and a sense of connection. Reflexology, through gentle touch, can build on this innate need and offer a range of potential benefits:

- **Soothing Colic and Discomfort:** Reflexology techniques applied to specific reflex points on the feet may help alleviate gas and digestive discomfort associated with colic.

- **Promoting Relaxation and Sleep:** The calming touch of reflexology can help soothe a fussy baby and encourage restful sleep.

- **Building a Bond:** Reflexology sessions can become a special bonding experience between parent and child.

Important Considerations:

- **Age Appropriateness:** Reflexology for babies is generally safe and well-tolerated, but it's best to start after the initial newborn fussiness subsides, typically around 6-8 weeks of age.

- **Consult a Pediatrician:** Always consult your pediatrician before starting any new therapy with your baby, including reflexology.

- **Less is More:** Sessions for babies should be brief, typically lasting 5-10 minutes. Focus on gentle strokes and light pressure.

Baby Reflexology Techniques:

Here are some basic reflexology techniques you can use with your baby:

- **The "I Love You" Stroke:** Starting at the base of the big toe, gently stroke upwards along the inner arch of the foot towards the heel. Repeat this motion 3-5 times on each foot, creating a heart shape with your thumb and index finger. This technique can be very calming and promote relaxation.

- **Solar Plexus Reflex:** Locate the solar plexus reflex on the sole of the foot, just below the base of the big toe. Apply gentle circular motions with your thumb for a few seconds on each foot. This reflex point is believed to influence the nervous system and promote relaxation.

- **Foot Rocking:** Gently cradle your baby's foot in your hand and rock it back and forth slowly. This can be a soothing technique, especially before bedtime.

Remember:

Always pay attention to your baby's cues. If they seem uncomfortable or fussy, stop the session. Reflexology should be a positive experience for both you and your baby.

A Gentle Journey Towards Well-being:

By incorporating these gentle reflexology techniques into your parenting routine, you can explore a natural approach to promoting your baby's well-being and fostering a loving bond through the power of touch. As your child grows, you can explore adapting reflexology techniques for their evolving needs, creating a foundation of self-care that can benefit them throughout their lives.

Providing Reflexology Care for Pregnancy and Postpartum Support

The journey of motherhood is a transformative experience, filled with joy, anticipation, and sometimes, physical discomfort. Reflexology offers a gentle and complementary approach to support women throughout pregnancy and the postpartum period. This chapter examines how reflexology can be adapted to address the unique needs of mothers-to-be and new mothers, fostering a sense of well-being throughout this remarkable life stage.

Understanding Reflexology During Pregnancy and Postpartum

Pregnancy and postpartum bring about a cascade of hormonal changes that affect the body in profound ways. Reflexology techniques can be tailored to address specific needs during each stage:

- **Pregnancy:** Reflexology can potentially help alleviate common pregnancy discomforts like nausea, morning sickness, backaches, and anxiety. It may also promote relaxation and improve sleep quality.

- **Postpartum:** During the postpartum period, reflexology can potentially aid in recovery from childbirth, support emotional well-being, and even promote lactation (breast milk production).

Important Considerations:

- **The First Trimester:** It's generally recommended to wait until the second trimester to begin reflexology sessions during pregnancy. This is due to the risk of stimulating uterine contractions in the early stages. Always consult a healthcare professional and a qualified prenatal reflexologist before starting reflexology while pregnant.

- **Communication is Key:** Open communication is crucial throughout pregnancy and postpartum. Discuss any concerns you have with your reflexologist and adjust pressure or techniques accordingly.

Reflexology Techniques for Pregnancy and Postpartum Support

Here are some reflexology techniques that can be adapted for pregnancy and postpartum support:

Pregnancy:

- **Solar Plexus Reflex:** Located on the sole of the foot, just below the diaphragm, the solar plexus reflex can be stimulated with gentle circular motions. This may promote relaxation and potentially alleviate nausea and anxiety.

- **Sacrum Reflex:** Found on the lower back of the foot, the sacrum reflex can be gently stimulated to potentially ease lower back pain, a common complaint during pregnancy.

- **Kidney Reflexes:** Located on the inner soles of the feet, the kidney reflexes can be stimulated with gentle strokes. This may support healthy fluid balance and potentially reduce swelling.

Postpartum:

- **Uterine Reflex:** Situated on the lower abdomen of the foot, the uterine reflex can be gently stimulated after childbirth to potentially aid in postpartum recovery. It's crucial to consult a qualified postpartum reflexologist for proper technique.

- **Spleen Reflex:** Found on the inner aspect of the foot, the spleen reflex can be stimulated to potentially enhance energy levels and promote emotional well-being, which can be challenged during the postpartum period.

- **Lactation Reflexes:** Several reflex points on the hands and feet are believed to correspond to lactation. Stimulating these points with a qualified reflexologist may potentially support breast milk production.

Remember:

Reflexology is a complementary therapy, not a replacement for medical care. Always consult your doctor or midwife for any health concerns you may have before or during pregnancy and postpartum.

A Journey of Nurturing Support

By incorporating reflexology sessions into your prenatal and postpartum care routine, you can potentially experience a greater sense of well-being throughout motherhood. This gentle touch can offer relief from physical discomfort, promote relaxation, and even strengthen the bond between mother and baby.

Considerations for Reflexology with Elderly Clients

The golden years hold immense wisdom and experience, but they can also be accompanied by physical limitations and age-related concerns. Reflexology offers a gentle and complementary approach to potentially support the well-being of elderly clients. Here, you'll explore the unique considerations for providing reflexology care to this cherished population.

Understanding the Needs of Elderly Clients:

The aging body presents unique challenges. Here's how reflexology can be adapted to address the specific needs of elderly clients:

- **Reduced Mobility:** Limited mobility can make it difficult for elderly clients to lie on a massage table. Consider offering reflexology sessions in a comfortable chair or while they're seated on the edge of the bed.

- **Thinning Skin:** As we age, our skin becomes thinner and more delicate. Utilize a lighter touch and adjust pressure according to the client's comfort level.

- **Pre-existing Conditions:** Many elderly clients have pre-existing health conditions. Consult with their doctor before starting reflexology sessions to ensure it's safe and appropriate.

Tailoring Reflexology Techniques for Elderly Clients

Here are some reflexology techniques that can be adapted for elderly clients:

- **Focus on Relaxation:** Prioritize techniques that promote relaxation and stress relief. Utilize gentle strokes on the solar plexus reflex (located on the sole of the foot, just below the diaphragm) and the head reflex points on the toes or instep.

- **Improved Circulation:** Stimulating circulation can potentially benefit elderly clients experiencing fatigue or aches and pains. Apply gentle strokes on the arch reflex (located on the sole of the foot) and consider incorporating foot soaks with essential oils like peppermint or rosemary before the session.

- **Promote Pain Management:** For targeted pain management, consult a reflexology chart to identify reflex points corresponding to specific areas of discomfort (e.g., knee pain, back pain). Utilize very gentle pressure or stroking techniques on these points.

Creating a Safe and Respectful Environment

Here are some additional considerations for creating a safe and respectful environment for elderly clients:

- **Open Communication:** Maintain open communication with your client. Ask about any pain or discomfort they experience and adjust pressure or techniques accordingly.

- **Warmth and Comfort:** Ensure the room is warm and well-lit. Provide pillows or blankets for additional comfort.

- **Respectful Touch:** Always ask permission before touching your client's feet. Use a gentle and respectful touch throughout the session.

- **Shorter Sessions:** Consider shorter reflexology sessions (around 15-20 minutes) for elderly clients, especially if they have limited attention spans or fatigue easily.

The Power of Human Connection

Reflexology for elderly clients goes beyond just the physical benefits. The human connection and gentle touch offered during a session can be deeply comforting and reduce feelings of isolation.

Remember:

Reflexology is a complementary therapy, not a substitute for medical care. Always consult with the client's doctor before starting reflexology sessions to ensure it's safe and appropriate

Integrating Reflexology into Your Daily Routine for Lasting Wellness

The human body is a magnificent machine, but even the most well-oiled machines benefit from regular maintenance. Reflexology offers a simple yet powerful tool you can integrate into your daily routine to promote lasting well-being. Here you will explore how to make reflexology a regular habit, allowing you to reap the potential benefits of this practice throughout your day.

The Power of Small, Consistent Steps

While some envision reflexology as hour-long spa sessions, the true magic lies in its accessibility. By incorporating short, self-administered reflexology techniques into your daily routine, you can unlock a sense of calm, manage stress, and potentially improve your overall well-being.

Simple Techniques for Daily Integration

Here are some easy-to-implement reflexology techniques you can incorporate into your day:

- **The Morning Boost:** Start your day with a five-minute foot massage. Focus on gentle strokes from the heel towards the toes, stimulating circulation and promoting wakefulness.

- **Desk Detox:** Combat afternoon slumps with a quick reflexology break at your desk. Apply gentle pressure to the solar plexus reflex (located on the sole of the foot, just below the diaphragm) for a few seconds to encourage relaxation.

- **Pre-Sleep Ritual:** Unwind before bed with a calming foot soak infused with essential oils like lavender or chamomile. Follow this with gentle reflexology strokes on the feet and ankles to promote relaxation and prepare your body for restful sleep.

- **The Power of Pairs:** If you live with a partner or close friend, consider incorporating reflexology into your bonding time. Take turns giving each other short foot massages, focusing on areas of tension or discomfort.

Beyond the Feet: Exploring Hand Reflexology

Reflexology isn't confined to the feet! The hands also hold a map to well-being. Here are some simple hand reflexology techniques you can try:

- **Headache Relief:** Locate the space between the thumb and index finger on your hand. Apply gentle pressure to this point for a few seconds on each hand for potential headache relief.

- **Digestive Ease:** The fleshy area at the base of the thumb on your hand is believed to correspond with the digestive system. Rub this area gently in circular motions for a few minutes to potentially soothe digestive discomfort.

Remember:

Consistency is key! By integrating short reflexology sessions into your daily routine, you can create a powerful self-care practice that supports your well-being over the long term.

Building a Personalized Reflexology Routine

The beauty of reflexology lies in its adaptability. Experiment with different techniques and find what works best for you. Pay attention to how your body responds and tailor your routine accordingly. There are also numerous reflexology resources available online and in libraries, offering a wealth of techniques you can explore.

Finding a Reflexology Practitioner and Continuing Your Journey

Your exploration of reflexology has opened a door to a world of potential benefits. Now you might be wondering, "How do I take the next step and experience reflexology firsthand?" These pages will guide you through finding a qualified reflexology practitioner and offers resources to continue your journey with this complementary therapy.

Finding the Perfect Fit: Selecting a Reflexology Practitioner

The key to a successful reflexology experience lies in finding a practitioner who aligns with your needs and preferences. Here are some tips to guide your search:

- **Seek Recommendations:** Talk to friends, family, or your healthcare professional for recommendations. Positive word-of-mouth referrals can be a great starting point.

- **Research Credentials:** Look for a practitioner who is certified by a reputable reflexology organization. This ensures they have received proper training and adhere to professional standards.

- **Consider Experience:** Experience can be valuable, but don't discount the skills of a newer practitioner. Read online reviews or testimonials to get a sense of their approach and client satisfaction.

- **Schedule a Consultation:** Many reflexology practitioners offer consultations before booking a session. This allows you to discuss your goals and expectations, and ensures you feel comfortable with the practitioner's approach.

Continuing Your Reflexology Journey

Once you've experienced reflexology, you might be eager to learn more and potentially incorporate self-reflexology techniques into your daily routine. Here are some resources to fuel your continued exploration:

- **Professional Associations:** Many reflexology associations offer educational resources for the public, including online articles, webinars, and workshops.

- **Books and Online Resources:** A wealth of books and online resources delve deeper into reflexology theory, techniques, and self-care practices. Explore libraries, bookstores, or reputable online sources for reliable information.

- **Workshops and Classes:** Consider enrolling in workshops or classes offered by qualified reflexology instructors. This allows you to learn new techniques and deepen your understanding of the practice in a hands-on environment.

Embrace the Power of Self-Care

Reflexology is a powerful tool for self-care, but it's just one piece of the puzzle. Consider incorporating other healthy habits into your routine, such as a balanced diet, regular exercise, and stress-management techniques. By embracing a holistic approach to well-being, you empower yourself to thrive and live your best life.

Remember:

The journey of well-being is a lifelong exploration. Finding a qualified reflexology practitioner and continuing your learning journey opens doors to new possibilities for managing stress, promoting relaxation, and nurturing your overall health. So, take that next step, embrace the power of self-care, and watch your well-being blossom

Conclusion

The world of reflexology is no longer a mystery. You've explored its potential benefits, learned about contraindications, and discovered how to adapt this practice for various populations. You've even gained valuable insights into creating a safe and rewarding experience, both for yourself and others.

This newfound knowledge empowers you to take an active role in your well-being. Whether you choose to explore self-reflexology techniques or seek the expertise of a qualified practitioner, reflexology offers a path towards a more balanced and relaxed you.

The human body is a magnificent instrument, and reflexology offers a gentle way to unlock its potential for healing and self-care. Don't let this knowledge gather dust on a shelf. Take action! Schedule a consultation, explore self-reflexology techniques, or share this knowledge with a loved one.

Remember, a healthier, happier you is just a step away. So, embark on this journey of self-discovery, and embrace the power of reflexology to transform your well-being.

Farewell, and best wishes on your path to a life filled with greater balance and vitality!

Appendix

Glossary of Reflexology Terms

This glossary provides definitions for some key terms you'll encounter in the world of reflexology:

- **Reflexology:** A complementary therapy that involves applying pressure to specific points on the feet and sometimes hands, believed to correspond with different organs and systems in the body.

- **Reflex Point:** A specific area on the foot or hand believed to be connected to an organ or system in the body.

- **Pressure:** The amount of force applied during a reflexology session. Pressure should be gentle to moderate, and adjusted based on the client's comfort level and needs.

- **Contraindication:** A condition or situation where reflexology is not recommended. Examples include certain medical conditions, pregnancy during the first trimester, and open wounds.

- **Client:** The individual receiving a reflexology session.

- **Practitioner:** A qualified professional trained in the practice of reflexology.

- **Self-reflexology:** The practice of applying reflexology techniques on oneself.

- **Relaxation:** A primary goal of reflexology, achieved by promoting the body's natural relaxation response.

- **Stress Management:** Reflexology can be a valuable tool for managing stress and promoting feelings of calmness.

- **Holistic:** A whole-body approach to health and well-being, which reflexology can support.

- **Circulation:** The movement of blood throughout the body. Reflexology may help improve circulation in the feet and potentially throughout the body.

- **Well-being:** A state of overall physical, mental, and emotional health. Reflexology can be a tool for promoting overall well-being.

Additional Terms You Might Encounter:

- **Meridians:** Lines of energy flow believed to exist in the body, with reflex points corresponding to specific meridians (traditional Chinese medicine concept).

- **Solar Plexus Reflex:** A reflex point located on the sole of the foot, believed to correspond with the solar plexus (a network of nerves in the upper abdomen) and potentially promote relaxation.

- **Spleen Reflex:** A reflex point located on the inner aspect of the foot, believed to correspond with the spleen and potentially support energy levels and emotional well-being.

This glossary is not exhaustive, but it provides a foundation for understanding the key terms used in reflexology. As you delve deeper into this practice, you'll encounter additional terminology specific to reflexology techniques and applications.

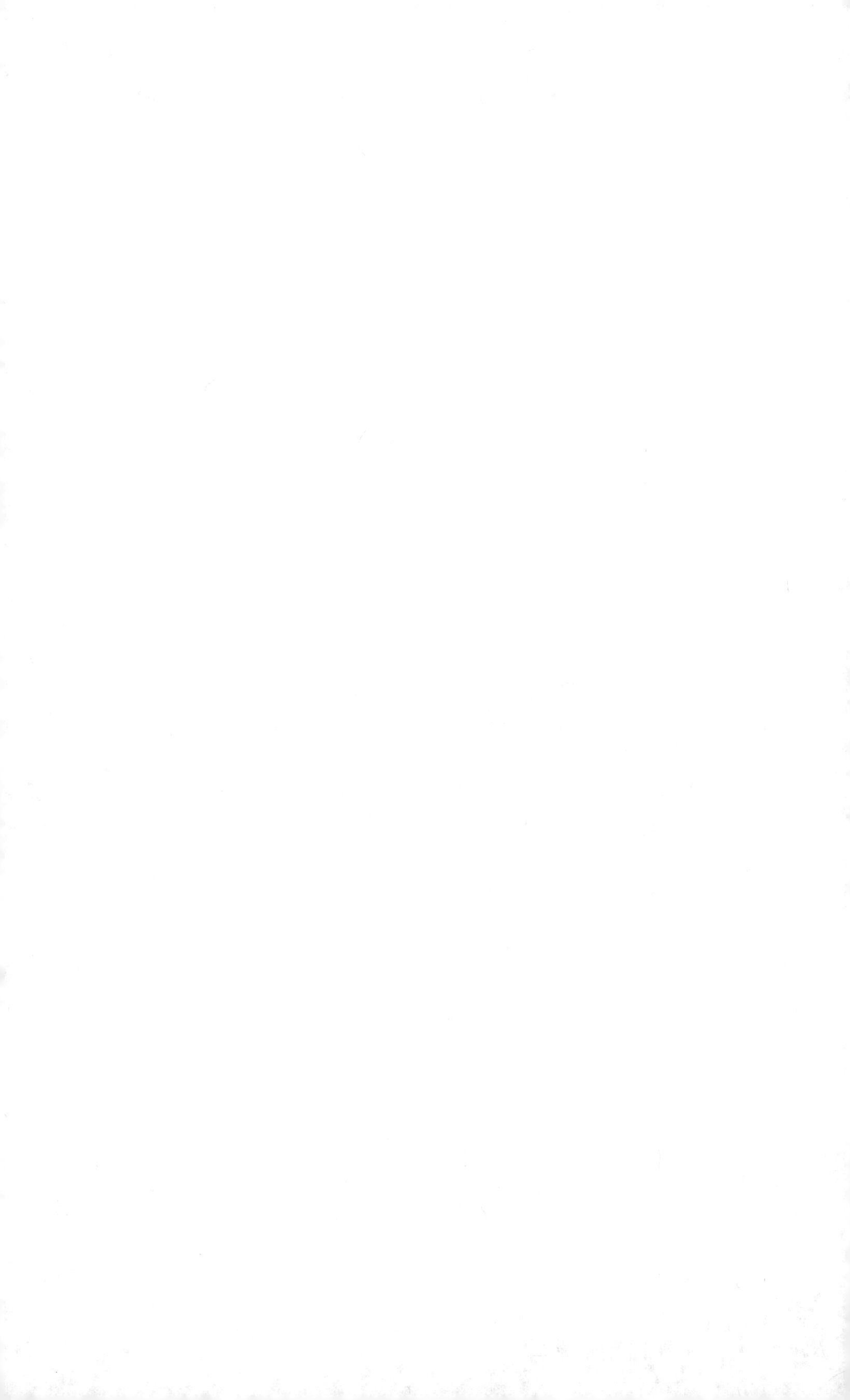